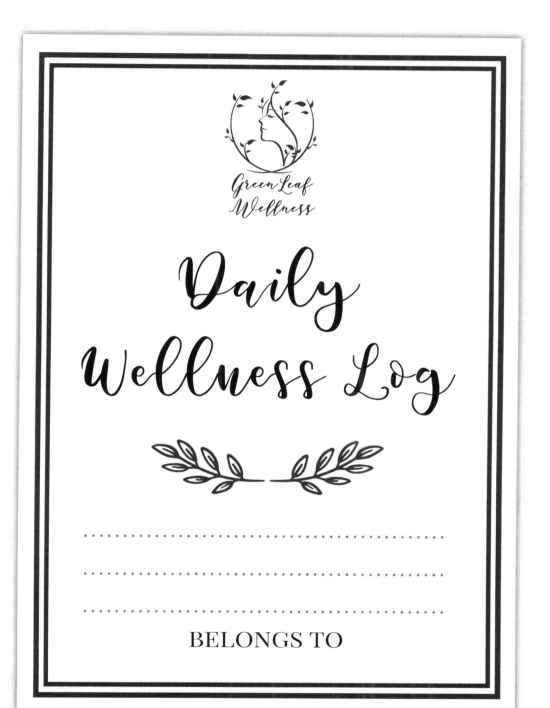

Green Leaf Wellness

Daily Wellness Log

....

....

....

BELONGS TO

Introduction

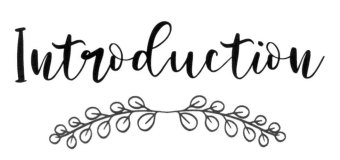

At **GreenLeaf Wellness**, we believe information can be a powerful tool - *especially* when it comes to our health and mental wellness!

We designed this book because we were personally fed up with trying to keep track of all our health symptoms either in our head or scattered throughout various notebooks and journals. We're still a bit old-fashioned in that we prefer to use good 'ol pen-and-paper. And none of the journals available on the market were what we wanted either. They were missing factors we thought were important to our health. And too many were a snooze fest to look at that we knew we wouldn't actually enjoy using them day after day, month after month. So we set out to create our own health tracker.

We wanted it to be a "one-stop shop" for women to record all their daily health information and to keep track of as many health-factors as possible. We also wanted it to be easy-to-use and pretty to look - which are both important factors in maintaining consistency in a tracking habit!

This ***Daily Wellness Log*** is the final result of all our efforts. If, like us, you've struggled with similar health tracking issues, we hope you find this journal to be the perfect solution for your health needs too!

In order to get the most benefit out of your ***Daily Wellness Log***, we recommend making it a habit to fill it out daily with as much information as possible. You may find it helpful to keep it with you wherever you go to jot information down as it happens. Or you can make a plan to grab a hot cup of soothing herbal tea and fill it out every evening as part of your bedtime ritual.

Ultimately though, this journal is **YOUR** journal. Do what feels right for you. The "wellness police" won't be after you if you don't fill it out every day. If you miss a day (*or two or a week*), or you just need to take a break from tracking, don't stress about it! Just continue where you left off when you're ready. And remember, this journal is meant to fit your own personal needs, so don't feel pressured to fill out everything. Just focus on filling out the parts that support your own personal health journey.

Wishing you well on your own wellness journey,
The GreenLeaf Wellness Team

How to Use this Book

Section 1

Date / Day of the Week / Weight / Temperature / Hours of Sleep / Sleep Quality

Daily Wellness Log Date: _____   S M T W Th F Sa

Weight:

Temperature:

Hours of Sleep
0 1 2 3 4 5 6 7 8 9 10 11 12+

Sleep Quality
☆ ☆ ☆ ☆ ☆

Date: Simply write in today's date here

Day of the Week: Circle/highlight the appropriate day of the week.

Weight: Record your weight here. Try to weigh yourself at the same time of day and wear the same of amount of clothing (*or none at all if that's how you roll*) for a true apples-to-apples comparison.

Temperature: This space is for keeping track of your basal body temperature (BBT) using a special thermometer to help you get an idea of when you're ovulating. For best results, take your BBT first thing after waking, before sitting upright, and while lying still in bed. You'll want to take it at the same time every day too. Be sure to jot down a note for any days that may have unreliable data due to illness, heavy drinking, jet lag, or changes in your sleeping patterns - which can all cause changes to your menstrual cycle.

Hours of Sleep: Circle/highlight the appropriate amount of hours you slept.

Sleep Quality: Color, circle or highlight the total number of stars that represent the quality of sleep. As a general guideline, use the following criteria to determine your number of stars:

1 star = Absolutely awful - didn't sleep a wink!

2 stars = Up & wandering around the house. I'm definitely going to need a nap later.

3 stars = Kept tossing & turning but eventually got some sleep.

4 stars = Slept through most of the night. Woke up once or twice, but fell right back to sleep.

5 stars = Slept completely through the night and feel well rested. Best sleep ever!

How to Use this Book cont.

Section 2
Weather / Temperature / Moon

⭐**4** **Weather and Temperature:** Some people (*raising our hands here*) are physically and mentally affected by the weather. Check each box that applies to the day's weather and temperature.

⭐**5** **Moon:** Some people are also impacted by the phases of the moon (*raising our hands here again*). Studies have shown the moon can impact our sleep. The scientific jury's still inconclusive though on it affecting other aspects of our health, like our mood and menstrual cycle. Best way to find out if you are personally affected by the moon is to keep track. Check the box for the day's phase of the moon.

Weather
- ☐ Sunny ☀
- ☐ Partly Cloudy ☁
- ☐ Cloudy ⛅
- ☐ Windy 🌬
- ☐ Stormy ⛈
- ☐ Light Rain 🌦
- ☐ Heavy Rain 🌧
- ☐ Light Snow 🌨
- ☐ Heavy Snow 🌨
- ☐ Other

⭐**4**

Temperature
- ☐ Hot
- ☐ Warm
- ☐ Cold
- ☐ Damp
- ☐ Comfortable

⭐**5**

Moon
- ☐ New Moon ●
- ☐ Waxing Crescent ●
- ☐ First Quarter ◐
- ☐ Waxing Gibbous ◑
- ☐ Full Moon ○
- ☐ Waning Gibbous ◑
- ☐ Third Quarter ◑
- ☐ Waning Crescent ●

Section 3
Mood / Water / Energy Level / Bowel Movement

⭐**6** **Mood:** Check each box that applies to the day's mood.

⭐**7** **Water:** Each water glass icon corresponds to 8 ounces (*or 1 cup*). Simply color, circle or highlight the number of water glass icons equal to how many ounces or cups you've consumed. A common suggestion for how much water to drink a day is eight-8oz glasses of water (*or 64 ounces total*). Your own personal hydration needs however are dependent on many factors such as physical activity, your weight, metabolism, etc. The best method to ensure you're properly hydrated during the day is to pay attention to your pee - it should be the color of lemonade (*aka slightly yellow*).

Mood
- ☐ Happy 🙂
- ☐ Calm 🙂
- ☐ Confident 😎
- ☐ Excited 😊
- ☐ Loving 😍
- ☐ Other
- ☐ Sad 🙁
- ☐ Angry 😠
- ☐ Anxious 😟
- ☐ Stressed 😣
- ☐ Self-Critical 😤
- ☐ Ti... 😫

⭐**6**

⭐**8**

⭐**7**

Water
☐☐☐☐☐☐☐☐

Energy Level
☆☆☆☆☆

⭐**9**

Bowel Movement

Constipation   Diarrhea

Type 1	Type 2	Type 3	Type 4	Type 5	Type 6	Type 7

Section 3 continued
Mood / Water / Energy Level / Bowel Movement

 Energy Level: Your energy levels naturally fluctuate during the day. This energy tracker is intended as a general overview or average of your day. Color, circle or highlight the total number of stars that represent your day's energy level. As a general guideline, use the following criteria to determine your number of stars:

1 star = I just can't deal with *anything* today.
2 stars = I barely dragged myself out of bed. Everything feels like a struggle today.
3 stars = It was hard to stay focused and I felt sluggish. Needed caffeine to get things going.
4 stars = I felt pretty good and got things done too.
5 stars = Bring it on! I'm ready to tackle anything!

 Bowel Movement: *Poop!* Nobody really likes to talk about it, but it's super-duper important. Your poop can say a lot about your health. If you aren't already taking a look at your stool, we highly recommend you start doing so (*and yes, it's kinda gross at first but you'll get over it - just think of it like a science experiment*). Check each box that corresponds to the day's type of bowel movement(s). We recommend the Bristol Stool Chart as a guideline for the types of stool you may experience. The guidelines are as follows:

Type 1 (Constipated) = Separate hard lumps that are hard to pass
(*like nuts*)

Type 2 (Slightly constipated) = Sausage-shaped but lumpy and somewhat difficult to pass
(*like a bunch of grapes*)

Type 3 (Normal) = Sausage-shaped with cracks on the surface that are easy to pass
(*like corn on the cob*)

Type 4 (Normal) = Sausage-or snake-shaped that are smooth, soft and easy to pass
(*like a banana*)

Type 5 (Lacking Fiber) = Soft blobs with clear-cut edges and easy to pass
(*like chicken nuggets*)

Type 6 (Slight Diarrhea) = Fluffy or mushy pieces with ragged edges
(*like porridge*)

Type 7 (Diarrhea) = Entirely liquid with no solid pieces (*like gravy*)

How to Use this Book cont.

Section 4
Medications / Vitamins

	Time	Description			Time	Description
Medications			⭐ 10	**Vitamins**		

Medications & Vitamins: Carefully complete these two sections as they may prove to be super-duper important to you later on. Write down the name of the drug and dosage strength (*such as 1,000mg or 500 IU*). Write down the time of day you took any medicine too. This is especially important if you have drugs that might interact with each other and you need to space them out appropriately throughout the day! Under the medications section, be sure to include any over-the-counter drugs along with any prescription medications you take during the day. And as for the vitamins section, make sure to include any herbal supplements you take too.

Section 5
Exercise

	Time	Intensity	⭐ 11	Activity
Exercise				

Exercise: Record the amount of time you were physically active along with the intensity level and brief description of the activity. For the intensity level, feel free to use the guidelines below as a reference:

Easy = Breathing is easy and I can carry on a conversation
Moderate = A bit out of breath, but can still carry on a conversation
Hard = Out of breath and I can only speak a word or two
Max = Seriously out of breath and I can't talk at all

How to Use this Book cont.

Section 6
Food and Drink

Breakfast	Lunch	Dinner	Snacks
		⭐12	

⭐12 **Food and Drink:** We're sure you've heard by now the sayings *"you are what you eat"* and *"food is medicine"* - and we couldn't agree more! Recording what you eat and drink is important, not just for weight loss purposes, but also to identify any potential food allergies. Record your food here (*and be sure to include any sample bites you might take throughout the day*). The level to which you record your food is entirely up to you. If you enjoy measuring your food and tracking your macros - you do you! If you simply want to jot down what you ate, that's okay too. Just try to write it all down.

Section 7
Menstrual Cycle Symptoms / Period

⭐13 **Menstrual Cycle Symptoms**

☐ Cramps ☐ Headache ☐ Backache ☐ Nausea ☐ Fatigue

☐ Tender Breasts ☐ Acne ☐ Bloating ☐ Cravings ☐ Insomnia

☐ Other

Physical Symptoms Log ⭐14

Period

☐ Spotting ☐ Light ☐ Medium ☐ Heavy

 ⭐13 **Menstrual Cycle Symptoms:** Check each box that applies to the day's menstrual cycle symptoms.

⭐14 **Period:** Check each box that applies to the day's period flow. As a general guideline, use the following criteria to determine your flow level:

Spotting = just a few drops of blood throughout the day
Light = Needing to change a low absorbency or regular tampon/pad 2 to 3 times per day
Medium = Needing to change a regular absorbency tampon/pad 4 to 6 times per day
Heavy = Needing to change a high absorbency tampon/pad every 3-4 hours

Section 7

Pain, Discomfort and Skin Changes

Pain, Discomfort and Skin Changes

(See the Pain Level Reference and/or Glossary for help in describing your symptoms)

Describe your symptoms, pain level and approximate time in the appropriate space below:

☐ Head / Ears / Eyes / Nose / Mouth

⭐ 16

_____

_____

_____

☐ Shoulders / Arms / Hands

_____

_____

_____

☐ Back

_____

_____

_____

☐ Lungs / Breathing (Respiratory)

_____

_____

_____

☐ Uterus / Vagina (Reproductive)

_____

_____

_____

☐ Other

_____

_____

_____

☐ Throat / Neck

_____

_____

_____

☐ Chest / Heart

_____

_____

_____

☐ Hips / Buttocks / Legs / Feet

_____

_____

_____

☐ Stomach / Abdomen (Digestive)

_____

_____

_____

☐ Skin

_____

_____

_____

Mark all the places on the diagram below that you are experiencing pain, discomfort, and/or skin changes:

Front

⭐ 15

Back

How to Use this Book cont.

Section 7 continued

Pain, Discomfort and/or Skin Changes

 Illustrated Body Diagram: Mark on the diagram where you are experiencing any aches, pains or skin changes as a visual reference for your symptoms.

 Symptom Description: Check each area that you've noticed a change or are experiencing any symptoms. In the space provided, briefly describe the specific symptom(s), pain level (if any), and time of day.

Pain Level Reference

As a guideline, feel free to use the following criteria to determine your pain level when writing out your description:

1 **Minor**	2 **Noticeable**	3 **Distressing**	4 **Very Distressing**
Very light pain (*like a mosquito bite*)	Very noticeable pain, but can still function okay (*like a deep paper cut*)	Strong, deep pain (*like a toothache or stubbing your toe*)	Strong, deep, piercing pain (*like a sprained ankle*)

5 **Intense**	6 **Utterly Horrible**	7 **Excruciating**
Strong, deep, piercing pain you can barely think straight (*like a migraine headache*)	Pain so intense you can't think straight at all (*like childbirth*)	Pain so intense you're likely to loose consciousness

Pain Glossary

If you're struggling to describe the type of pain or discomfort you're feeling, below are a list of words to help get you started:

shooting	cramping	stinging	pinching	squeezing	shooting
stabbing	dull	piercing	tingling	itchy	stinging
burning	numbness	knot-like	coldness	crushing	gnawing
aching	pins and needles	tender	searing	nauseating	spreading
throbbing	pricking	radiating	wrenching	blinding	splitting

Daily Wellness Log Example Page

Daily Wellness Log   Date: 1/16/20   S M T W (Th) F Sa

Weight: 168.2 lbs
Temperature: 98.6°F

Hours of Sleep
0 1 2 3 4 5 (6) 7 8 9 10 11 12+

Sleep Quality
★★★☆☆

Weather
- [ ] Sunny ☀
- [ ] Partly Cloudy ⛅
- [x] Cloudy ⛅
- [x] Windy
- [ ] Stormy
- [ ] Light Rain
- [x] Heavy Rain
- [ ] Light Snow
- [ ] Heavy Snow
- [ ] Other

Mood
- [ ] Happy ☺
- [ ] Calm ☺
- [ ] Confident 😎
- [ ] Excited
- [ ] Loving 😍
- [x] Other Irritable
- [ ] Sad
- [ ] Angry
- [x] Anxious
- [ ] Stressed
- [x] Self-Critical
- [x] Tired

Temperature
- [ ] Hot
- [ ] Warm
- [x] Cold
- [x] Damp
- [ ] Comfortable

Water
(glasses: 4 filled, 3 empty)

Energy Level
★★★☆☆

Moon
- [ ] New Moon
- [ ] Waxing Crescent
- [ ] First Quarter
- [ ] Waxing Gibbous
- [ ] Full Moon
- [ ] Waning Gibbous
- [x] Third Quarter
- [ ] Waning Crescent

Bowel Movement
Constipation   Diarrhea
Type 1   Type 2   (Type 3)   Type 4   Type 5   Type 6   Type 7

Medications

Time	Description
5:30am	thyroid (100mcg levothyroxine)
4:00pm	advil (400mg)

Vitamins

Time	Description
6:00pm	women's multivitamin
"	vitamin D (1,000 IU)
"	fish oil (2,400 mg)
"	probiotic (80b CFU)

Exercise

Time	Intensity	Activity
30m	Easy	1.5 mile walk on treadmill @ lunch
30m	Easy	evening bedtime yoga + stretching session

Breakfast
* mushroom, spinach & egg quiche
* 2 cups coffee w/ cream & sugar

Lunch
* green goddess salad (starbucks)
* grande london fog (starbucks)

Dinner
* chicken alfredo pasta
* caesar salad (side)
* 3 pieces of garlic bread
* glass of chardonnay

Snacks
* handful of almonds
* carrot sticks + garlic hummus

Physical Symptoms Log Example Page

Menstrual Cycle Symptoms

- [ ] Cramps
- [✓] Headache
- [ ] Backache
- [ ] Nausea
- [ ] Fatigue
- [✓] Tender Breasts
- [✓] Acne
- [ ] Bloating
- [ ] Cravings
- [ ] Insomnia
- [ ] Other

Physical Symptoms Log

Period

- [ ] Spotting
- [ ] Light
- [ ] Medium
- [ ] Heavy

Pain, Discomfort and Skin Changes

(See the Pain Level Reference and/or Glossary for help in describing your symptoms)

Describe your symptoms, pain level and approximate time in the appropriate space below:

[✓] Head / Ears / Eyes / Nose / Mouth
throbbing headache @ 3:20pm
(level 3), took some advil;
on left side behind eye

[ ] Throat / Neck

[ ] Shoulders / Arms / Hands

[ ] Chest / Heart

[✓] Back
aching lower back (level 2)
throughout day; applied
heating pad

[ ] Hips / Buttocks / Legs / Feet

[ ] Lungs / Breathing (Respiratory)

[ ] Stomach / Abdomen (Digestive)

[✓] Uterus / Vagina (Reproductive)
brown discharge

[✓] Skin
cystic acne on chin
(level 2); left side

[ ] Other

Mark all the places on the diagram below that you are experiencing pain, discomfort, and/or skin changes:

headache   acne

Front

lower back pain   discharge

Back

Notes
should be starting period any day now. Feeling anxious about big meeting next week. Felt cranky at the smallest things today too.

Daily Wellness Log

Date: _____   S M T W Th F Sa

Weight: _____
Temperature: _____

Hours of Sleep

0 1 2 3 4 5 6 7 8 9 10 11 12+

Sleep Quality

☆ ☆ ☆ ☆ ☆

Weather

- ☐ Sunny ☀
- ☐ Partly Cloudy ☁
- ☐ Cloudy ⛅
- ☐ Windy 🌬
- ☐ Stormy ⛈
- ☐ Light Rain 🌦
- ☐ Heavy Rain 🌧
- ☐ Light Snow 🌨
- ☐ Heavy Snow 🌨
- ☐ Other ....

Mood

- ☐ Happy ☺
- ☐ Calm ☺
- ☐ Confident 😎
- ☐ Excited 😀
- ☐ Loving 😍
- ☐ Other ....
- ☐ Sad ☹
- ☐ Angry 😠
- ☐ Anxious 😟
- ☐ Stressed 😖
- ☐ Self-Critical 😈
- ☐ Tired 😫

Temperature

☐ Hot   ☐ Warm   ☐ Cold   ☐ Damp   ☐ Comfortable

Water

▽ ▽ ▽ ▽ ▽ ▽ ▽ ▽

Energy Level

☆ ☆ ☆ ☆ ☆

Moon

- ☐ New Moon ●
- ☐ Waxing Crescent ◐
- ☐ First Quarter ◑
- ☐ Waxing Gibbous ◑
- ☐ Full Moon ○
- ☐ Waning Gibbous ◑
- ☐ Third Quarter ◐
- ☐ Waning Crescent ◐

Bowel Movement

Constipation   *Diarrhea*

Type 1	Type 2	Type 3	Type 4	Type 5	Type 6	Type 7

Medications

Time	Description

Vitamins

Time	Description

Exercise

Time	Intensity	Activity

Breakfast

Lunch

Dinner

Snacks

Menstrual Cycle Symptoms

☐ Cramps ☐ Headache ☐ Backache ☐ Nausea ☐ Fatigue

☐ Tender Breasts ☐ Acne ☐ Bloating ☐ Cravings ☐ Insomnia

☐ Other ....

Physical Symptoms Log

Period

☐ Spotting ☐ Light ☐ Medium ☐ Heavy

Pain, Discomfort and Skin Changes

(See the Pain Level Reference and/or Glossary for help in describing your symptoms)

Describe your symptoms, pain level and approximate time in the appropriate space below:

☐ Head / Ears / Eyes / Nose / Mouth
_____
_____
_____

☐ Shoulders / Arms / Hands
_____
_____

☐ Back
_____
_____
_____

☐ Lungs / Breathing (Respiratory)
_____
_____

☐ Uterus / Vagina (Reproductive)
_____
_____

☐ Other
_____
_____

☐ Throat / Neck
_____
_____

☐ Chest / Heart
_____
_____
_____

☐ Hips / Buttocks / Legs / Feet
_____
_____
_____

☐ Stomach / Abdomen (Digestive)
_____
_____

☐ Skin
_____
_____

Mark all the places on the diagram below that you are experiencing pain, discomfort, and/or skin changes:

Front

Back

Notes
_____
_____
_____
_____

Daily Wellness Log

Date: ....   S M T W Th F Sa

Weight: _____
Temperature: _____

Hours of Sleep

0 1 2 3 4 5 6 7 8 9 10 11 12+

Sleep Quality

☆ ☆ ☆ ☆ ☆

Weather

- [ ] Sunny ☀
- [ ] Partly Cloudy ☁
- [ ] Cloudy ⛅
- [ ] Windy 🌬
- [ ] Stormy ⛈
- [ ] Light Rain 🌦
- [ ] Heavy Rain 🌧
- [ ] Light Snow 🌨
- [ ] Heavy Snow 🌨
- [ ] Other ....

Mood

- [ ] Happy ☺
- [ ] Calm ☺
- [ ] Confident 😎
- [ ] Excited ☺
- [ ] Loving 😍
- [ ] Other
- [ ] Sad ☹
- [ ] Angry 😠
- [ ] Anxious 😟
- [ ] Stressed 😖
- [ ] Self-Critical 😡
- [ ] Tired 😫

Temperature

[ ] Hot   [ ] Warm   [ ] Cold   [ ] Damp   [ ] Comfortable

Water

🥤 🥤 🥤 🥤 🥤 🥤 🥤 🥤

Energy Level

☆ ☆ ☆ ☆ ☆

Moon

- [ ] New Moon ●
- [ ] Waxing Crescent ●
- [ ] First Quarter ◑
- [ ] Waxing Gibbous ◑
- [ ] Full Moon ○
- [ ] Waning Gibbous ◐
- [ ] Third Quarter ◐
- [ ] Waning Crescent ◐

Bowel Movement

Constipation   *Diarrhea*

Type 1	Type 2	Type 3	Type 4	Type 5	Type 6	Type 7

Medications

Time	Description

Vitamins

Time	Description

Exercise

Time	Intensity	Activity

Breakfast

Lunch

Dinner

Snacks

Menstrual Cycle Symptoms

- [ ] Cramps
- [ ] Headache
- [ ] Backache
- [ ] Nausea
- [ ] Fatigue
- [ ] Tender Breasts
- [ ] Acne
- [ ] Bloating
- [ ] Cravings
- [ ] Insomnia
- [ ] Other

Physical Symptoms Log

Period

- [ ] Spotting
- [ ] Light
- [ ] Medium
- [ ] Heavy

Pain, Discomfort and Skin Changes

(See the Pain Level Reference and/or Glossary for help in describing your symptoms)

Describe your symptoms, pain level and approximate time in the appropriate space below:

- [ ] Head / Ears / Eyes / Nose / Mouth
  _____
  _____
  _____

- [ ] Throat / Neck
  _____
  _____

- [ ] Shoulders / Arms / Hands
  _____
  _____

- [ ] Chest / Heart
  _____
  _____

- [ ] Back
  _____
  _____
  _____

- [ ] Hips / Buttocks / Legs / Feet
  _____
  _____
  _____

- [ ] Lungs / Breathing (Respiratory)
  _____
  _____

- [ ] Stomach / Abdomen (Digestive)
  _____
  _____

- [ ] Uterus / Vagina (Reproductive)
  _____
  _____

- [ ] Skin
  _____
  _____

- [ ] Other
  _____
  _____
  _____

Mark all the places on the diagram below that you are experiencing pain, discomfort, and/or skin changes:

Front

Back

Notes
_____
_____
_____
_____
_____

Daily Wellness Log

Date: ....   S   M   T   W   Th   F   Sa

Weight:
Temperature:

Hours of Sleep

0   1   2   3   4   5   6   7   8   9   10   11   12+

Sleep Quality

☆ ☆ ☆ ☆ ☆

Weather

- [ ] Sunny ☀
- [ ] Partly Cloudy ☁
- [ ] Cloudy ⛅
- [ ] Windy 🌬
- [ ] Stormy ⛈
- [ ] Light Rain 🌧
- [ ] Heavy Rain 🌧
- [ ] Light Snow 🌨
- [ ] Heavy Snow ❄
- [ ] Other ....

Mood

- [ ] Happy 🙂
- [ ] Calm 🙂
- [ ] Confident 😎
- [ ] Excited 😄
- [ ] Loving 😍
- [ ] Other
- [ ] Sad ☹
- [ ] Angry 😠
- [ ] Anxious 😧
- [ ] Stressed 😖
- [ ] Self-Critical 😈
- [ ] Tired 😣

Temperature

- [ ] Hot
- [ ] Warm
- [ ] Cold
- [ ] Damp
- [ ] Comfortable

Water

🥛 🥛 🥛 🥛 🥛 🥛 🥛 🥛

Energy Level

☆ ☆ ☆ ☆ ☆

Moon

- [ ] New Moon ●
- [ ] Waxing Crescent ●
- [ ] First Quarter ◐
- [ ] Waxing Gibbous ◑
- [ ] Full Moon ○
- [ ] Waning Gibbous ◔
- [ ] Third Quarter ◑
- [ ] Waning Crescent ◐

Bowel Movement

Constipation   *Diarrhea*

Type 1	Type 2	Type 3	Type 4	Type 5	Type 6	Type 7

Medications

Time	Description

Vitamins

Time	Description

Exercise

Time	Intensity	Activity

Breakfast

Lunch

Dinner

Snacks

Menstrual Cycle Symptoms

- [ ] Cramps
- [ ] Headache
- [ ] Backache
- [ ] Nausea
- [ ] Fatigue
- [ ] Tender Breasts
- [ ] Acne
- [ ] Bloating
- [ ] Cravings
- [ ] Insomnia
- [ ] Other

Physical Symptoms Log

Period

- [ ] Spotting
- [ ] Light
- [ ] Medium
- [ ] Heavy

Pain, Discomfort and Skin Changes

(See the Pain Level Reference and/or Glossary for help in describing your symptoms)

Describe your symptoms, pain level and approximate time in the appropriate space below:

- [ ] Head / Ears / Eyes / Nose / Mouth

- [ ] Throat / Neck

- [ ] Shoulders / Arms / Hands

- [ ] Chest / Heart

- [ ] Back

- [ ] Hips / Buttocks / Legs / Feet

- [ ] Lungs / Breathing (Respiratory)

- [ ] Stomach / Abdomen (Digestive)

- [ ] Uterus / Vagina (Reproductive)

- [ ] Skin

- [ ] Other

Mark all the places on the diagram below that you are experiencing pain, discomfort, and/or skin changes:

Front

Back

Notes

Daily Wellness Log

Date: ....   S   M   T   W   Th   F   Sa

Weight:

Temperature:

Hours of Sleep

0   1   2   3   4   5   6   7   8   9   10   11   12+

Sleep Quality

☆ ☆ ☆ ☆ ☆

Weather

- [ ] Sunny ☀
- [ ] Partly Cloudy ☁
- [ ] Cloudy ⛅
- [ ] Windy 🌬
- [ ] Stormy ⛈
- [ ] Light Rain 🌧
- [ ] Heavy Rain 🌧
- [ ] Light Snow 🌨
- [ ] Heavy Snow 🌨
- [ ] Other ....

Temperature

- [ ] Hot
- [ ] Warm
- [ ] Cold
- [ ] Damp
- [ ] Comfortable

Moon

- [ ] New Moon ●
- [ ] Waxing Crescent ◔
- [ ] First Quarter ◑
- [ ] Waxing Gibbous ◕
- [ ] Full Moon ○
- [ ] Waning Gibbous ◔
- [ ] Third Quarter ◐
- [ ] Waning Crescent ◕

Mood

- [ ] Happy 🙂
- [ ] Calm 🙂
- [ ] Confident 😎
- [ ] Excited 😄
- [ ] Loving 😍
- [ ] Other
- [ ] Sad ☹
- [ ] Angry 😠
- [ ] Anxious 😧
- [ ] Stressed 😖
- [ ] Self-Critical 😡
- [ ] Tired 😫

Water

🥛 🥛 🥛 🥛 🥛 🥛 🥛 🥛

Energy Level

☆ ☆ ☆ ☆ ☆

Bowel Movement

Constipation   *Diarrhea*

Type 1	Type 2	Type 3	Type 4	Type 5	Type 6	Type 7

Medications

Time	Description

Vitamins

Time	Description

Exercise

Time	Intensity	Activity

Breakfast

Lunch

Dinner

Snacks

Menstrual Cycle Symptoms

- [ ] Cramps
- [ ] Headache
- [ ] Backache
- [ ] Nausea
- [ ] Fatigue
- [ ] Tender Breasts
- [ ] Acne
- [ ] Bloating
- [ ] Cravings
- [ ] Insomnia
- [ ] Other

Physical Symptoms Log

Period

- [ ] Spotting
- [ ] Light
- [ ] Medium
- [ ] Heavy

Pain, Discomfort and Skin Changes

(See the Pain Level Reference and/or Glossary for help in describing your symptoms)

Describe your symptoms, pain level and approximate time in the appropriate space below:

- [ ] Head / Ears / Eyes / Nose / Mouth
_____
_____
_____

- [ ] Throat / Neck
_____
_____
_____

- [ ] Shoulders / Arms / Hands
_____
_____
_____

- [ ] Chest / Heart
_____
_____
_____

- [ ] Back
_____
_____
_____

- [ ] Hips / Buttocks / Legs / Feet
_____
_____
_____

- [ ] Lungs / Breathing (Respiratory)
_____
_____
_____

- [ ] Stomach / Abdomen (Digestive)
_____
_____
_____

- [ ] Uterus / Vagina (Reproductive)
_____
_____
_____

- [ ] Skin
_____
_____
_____

- [ ] Other
_____
_____
_____

Mark all the places on the diagram below that you are experiencing pain, discomfort, and/or skin changes:

Front

Back

Notes
_____
_____
_____
_____

Daily Wellness Log

Date: ....

S M T W Th F Sa

Weight:
Temperature:

Hours of Sleep

0 1 2 3 4 5 6 7 8 9 10 11 12+

Sleep Quality

☆ ☆ ☆ ☆ ☆

Weather

- [ ] Sunny ☀
- [ ] Partly Cloudy ☁
- [ ] Cloudy ⛅
- [ ] Windy 🌬
- [ ] Stormy ⛈
- [ ] Light Rain 🌦
- [ ] Heavy Rain 🌧
- [ ] Light Snow 🌨
- [ ] Heavy Snow 🌨
- [ ] Other ....

Mood

- [ ] Happy 🙂
- [ ] Calm 🙂
- [ ] Confident 😎
- [ ] Excited 😃
- [ ] Loving 😍
- [ ] Other
- [ ] Sad ☹
- [ ] Angry 😠
- [ ] Anxious 😟
- [ ] Stressed 😣
- [ ] Self-Critical 😈
- [ ] Tired 😫

Temperature

- [ ] Hot
- [ ] Warm
- [ ] Cold
- [ ] Damp
- [ ] Comfortable

Water

⊔ ⊔ ⊔ ⊔ ⊔ ⊔ ⊔ ⊔

Energy Level

☆ ☆ ☆ ☆ ☆

Moon

- [ ] New Moon ●
- [ ] Waxing Crescent ◗
- [ ] First Quarter ◑
- [ ] Waxing Gibbous ◖
- [ ] Full Moon ○
- [ ] Waning Gibbous ◐
- [ ] Third Quarter ◐
- [ ] Waning Crescent ◖

Bowel Movement

Constipation   *Diarrhea*

Type 1	Type 2	Type 3	Type 4	Type 5	Type 6	Type 7

Medications

Time	Description

Vitamins

Time	Description

Exercise

Time	Intensity	Activity

Breakfast

Lunch

Dinner

Snacks

Menstrual Cycle Symptoms

- [ ] Cramps
- [ ] Headache
- [ ] Backache
- [ ] Nausea
- [ ] Fatigue
- [ ] Tender Breasts
- [ ] Acne
- [ ] Bloating
- [ ] Cravings
- [ ] Insomnia
- [ ] Other

Physical Symptoms Log

Period

- [ ] Spotting
- [ ] Light
- [ ] Medium
- [ ] Heavy

Pain, Discomfort and Skin Changes

(See the Pain Level Reference and/or Glossary for help in describing your symptoms)

Describe your symptoms, pain level and approximate time in the appropriate space below:

- [ ] Head / Ears / Eyes / Nose / Mouth
- [ ] Throat / Neck
- [ ] Shoulders / Arms / Hands
- [ ] Chest / Heart
- [ ] Back
- [ ] Hips / Buttocks / Legs / Feet
- [ ] Lungs / Breathing (Respiratory)
- [ ] Stomach / Abdomen (Digestive)
- [ ] Uterus / Vagina (Reproductive)
- [ ] Skin
- [ ] Other

Mark all the places on the diagram below that you are experiencing pain, discomfort, and/or skin changes:

Front

Back

Notes

Daily Wellness Log

Date: .... S M T W Th F Sa

Weight:
Temperature:

Hours of Sleep

0 1 2 3 4 5 6 7 8 9 10 11 12+

Sleep Quality

☆ ☆ ☆ ☆ ☆

Weather

- ☐ Sunny ☀
- ☐ Partly Cloudy ☁
- ☐ Cloudy ⛅
- ☐ Windy 🌬
- ☐ Stormy ⛈
- ☐ Light Rain 🌦
- ☐ Heavy Rain 🌧
- ☐ Light Snow 🌨
- ☐ Heavy Snow 🌨
- ☐ Other

Mood

- ☐ Happy ☺
- ☐ Calm ☺
- ☐ Confident 😎
- ☐ Excited 🙂
- ☐ Loving 😍
- ☐ Other
- ☐ Sad ☹
- ☐ Angry 😠
- ☐ Anxious 😧
- ☐ Stressed 😖
- ☐ Self-Critical 😠
- ☐ Tired 😫

Temperature

☐ Hot ☐ Warm ☐ Cold ☐ Damp ☐ Comfortable

Water

🥛 🥛 🥛 🥛 🥛 🥛 🥛 🥛

Energy Level

☆ ☆ ☆ ☆ ☆

Moon

- ☐ New Moon ●
- ☐ Waxing Crescent ◗
- ☐ First Quarter ◑
- ☐ Waxing Gibbous ◑
- ☐ Full Moon ○
- ☐ Waning Gibbous ◐
- ☐ Third Quarter ◐
- ☐ Waning Crescent ◕

Bowel Movement

Constipation   *Diarrhea*

Type 1	Type 2	Type 3	Type 4	Type 5	Type 6	Type 7

Medications

Time	Description

Vitamins

Time	Description

Exercise

Time	Intensity	Activity

Breakfast

Lunch

Dinner

Snacks

Menstrual Cycle Symptoms

- [ ] Cramps
- [ ] Headache
- [ ] Backache
- [ ] Nausea
- [ ] Fatigue
- [ ] Tender Breasts
- [ ] Acne
- [ ] Bloating
- [ ] Cravings
- [ ] Insomnia
- [ ] Other

Physical Symptoms Log

Period

- [ ] Spotting
- [ ] Light
- [ ] Medium
- [ ] Heavy

Pain, Discomfort and Skin Changes

(See the Pain Level Reference and/or Glossary for help in describing your symptoms)

Describe your symptoms, pain level and approximate time in the appropriate space below:

- [ ] Head / Ears / Eyes / Nose / Mouth

_____
_____

- [ ] Shoulders / Arms / Hands

_____
_____
_____

- [ ] Back

_____
_____
_____

- [ ] Lungs / Breathing (Respiratory)

_____
_____
_____

- [ ] Uterus / Vagina (Reproductive)

_____
_____
_____

- [ ] Other

_____
_____
_____

- [ ] Throat / Neck

_____
_____

- [ ] Chest / Heart

_____
_____
_____

- [ ] Hips / Buttocks / Legs / Feet

_____
_____
_____

- [ ] Stomach / Abdomen (Digestive)

_____
_____
_____

- [ ] Skin

_____
_____
_____

Mark all the places on the diagram below that you are experiencing pain, discomfort, and/or skin changes:

Front

Back

Notes

_____
_____
_____
_____

Daily Wellness Log

Date: .... 　　S　M　T　W　Th　F　Sa

Weight: _____
Temperature: _____

Hours of Sleep

0　1　2　3　4　5　6　7　8　9　10　11　12+

Sleep Quality

☆ ☆ ☆ ☆ ☆

Weather

- [ ] Sunny ☀
- [ ] Partly Cloudy ☁
- [ ] Cloudy ⛅
- [ ] Windy 🌬
- [ ] Stormy ⛈
- [ ] Light Rain 🌦
- [ ] Heavy Rain 🌧
- [ ] Light Snow 🌨
- [ ] Heavy Snow 🌨
- [ ] Other _____

Mood

- [ ] Happy 🙂
- [ ] Calm 🙂
- [ ] Confident 😎
- [ ] Excited 😃
- [ ] Loving 😍
- [ ] Other _____
- [ ] Sad ☹
- [ ] Angry 😠
- [ ] Anxious 😣
- [ ] Stressed 😖
- [ ] Self-Critical 😡
- [ ] Tired 😫

Temperature

- [ ] Hot
- [ ] Warm
- [ ] Cold
- [ ] Damp
- [ ] Comfortable

Water

🥛 🥛 🥛 🥛 🥛 🥛 🥛 🥛

Energy Level

☆ ☆ ☆ ☆ ☆

Moon

- [ ] New Moon ●
- [ ] Waxing Crescent ●
- [ ] First Quarter ◑
- [ ] Waxing Gibbous ◑
- [ ] Full Moon ○
- [ ] Waning Gibbous ◐
- [ ] Third Quarter ◐
- [ ] Waning Crescent ◐

Bowel Movement

Constipation　　　　　　　　　　　　　*Diarrhea*

Type 1	Type 2	Type 3	Type 4	Type 5	Type 6	Type 7

Medications

Time	Description

Vitamins

Time	Description

Exercise

Time	Intensity	Activity

Breakfast

Lunch

Dinner

Snacks

Menstrual Cycle Symptoms

- [ ] Cramps
- [ ] Headache
- [ ] Backache
- [ ] Nausea
- [ ] Fatigue
- [ ] Tender Breasts
- [ ] Acne
- [ ] Bloating
- [ ] Cravings
- [ ] Insomnia
- [ ] Other

Physical Symptoms Log

Period

- [ ] Spotting
- [ ] Light
- [ ] Medium
- [ ] Heavy

Pain, Discomfort and Skin Changes

(See the Pain Level Reference and/or Glossary for help in describing your symptoms)

Describe your symptoms, pain level and approximate time in the appropriate space below:

- [ ] Head / Ears / Eyes / Nose / Mouth
- [ ] Throat / Neck
- [ ] Shoulders / Arms / Hands
- [ ] Chest / Heart
- [ ] Back
- [ ] Hips / Buttocks / Legs / Feet
- [ ] Lungs / Breathing (Respiratory)
- [ ] Stomach / Abdomen (Digestive)
- [ ] Uterus / Vagina (Reproductive)
- [ ] Skin
- [ ] Other

Mark all the places on the diagram below that you are experiencing pain, discomfort, and/or skin changes:

Front

Back

Notes

Daily Wellness Log

Date: ....   S   M   T   W   Th   F   Sa

Weight:

Temperature:

Hours of Sleep

0   1   2   3   4   5   6   7   8   9   10   11   12+

Sleep Quality

☆ ☆ ☆ ☆ ☆

Weather

- [ ] Sunny ☀
- [ ] Partly Cloudy ⛅
- [ ] Cloudy ⛅
- [ ] Windy ☁
- [ ] Stormy ⛈
- [ ] Light Rain 🌧
- [ ] Heavy Rain 🌧
- [ ] Light Snow 🌨
- [ ] Heavy Snow 🌨
- [ ] Other ....

Mood

- [ ] Happy ☺
- [ ] Calm ☺
- [ ] Confident 😎
- [ ] Excited 😀
- [ ] Loving 😍
- [ ] Other
- [ ] Sad ☹
- [ ] Angry 😠
- [ ] Anxious 😣
- [ ] Stressed 😖
- [ ] Self-Critical 😡
- [ ] Tired 😫

Temperature

- [ ] Hot
- [ ] Warm
- [ ] Cold
- [ ] Damp
- [ ] Comfortable

Water

🥤 🥤 🥤 🥤 🥤 🥤 🥤 🥤

Energy Level

☆ ☆ ☆ ☆ ☆

Moon

- [ ] New Moon ●
- [ ] Waxing Crescent ●
- [ ] First Quarter ◑
- [ ] Waxing Gibbous ◐
- [ ] Full Moon ○
- [ ] Waning Gibbous ◔
- [ ] Third Quarter ◑
- [ ] Waning Crescent ◐

Bowel Movement

Constipation   *Diarrhea*

Type 1	Type 2	Type 3	Type 4	Type 5	Type 6	Type 7

Medications

Time	Description

Vitamins

Time	Description

Exercise

Time	Intensity	Activity

Breakfast

Lunch

Dinner

Snacks

Menstrual Cycle Symptoms

- [ ] Cramps
- [ ] Headache
- [ ] Backache
- [ ] Nausea
- [ ] Fatigue
- [ ] Tender Breasts
- [ ] Acne
- [ ] Bloating
- [ ] Cravings
- [ ] Insomnia
- [ ] Other

Physical Symptoms Log

Period

- [ ] Spotting
- [ ] Light
- [ ] Medium
- [ ] Heavy

Pain, Discomfort and Skin Changes

(See the Pain Level Reference and/or Glossary for help in describing your symptoms)

Describe your symptoms, pain level and approximate time in the appropriate space below:

- [ ] Head / Ears / Eyes / Nose / Mouth
- [ ] Throat / Neck
- [ ] Shoulders / Arms / Hands
- [ ] Chest / Heart
- [ ] Back
- [ ] Hips / Buttocks / Legs / Feet
- [ ] Lungs / Breathing (Respiratory)
- [ ] Stomach / Abdomen (Digestive)
- [ ] Uterus / Vagina (Reproductive)
- [ ] Skin
- [ ] Other

Mark all the places on the diagram below that you are experiencing pain, discomfort, and/or skin changes:

Front

Back

Notes

Daily Wellness Log

Date: ....   S   M   T   W   Th   F   Sa

Weight: _____
Temperature: _____

Hours of Sleep

0   1   2   3   4   5   6   7   8   9   10   11   12+

Sleep Quality

☆ ☆ ☆ ☆ ☆

Weather

- ☐ Sunny ☀
- ☐ Partly Cloudy ☁
- ☐ Cloudy ⛅
- ☐ Windy 🌬
- ☐ Stormy ⛈
- ☐ Light Rain 🌧
- ☐ Heavy Rain 🌧
- ☐ Light Snow 🌨
- ☐ Heavy Snow 🌨
- ☐ Other _____

Mood

- ☐ Happy ☺
- ☐ Calm ☺
- ☐ Confident 😎
- ☐ Excited ☺
- ☐ Loving 😍
- ☐ Other
- ☐ Sad ☹
- ☐ Angry 😠
- ☐ Anxious 😨
- ☐ Stressed 😣
- ☐ Self-Critical 😡
- ☐ Tired 😫

Temperature

☐ Hot   ☐ Warm   ☐ Cold   ☐ Damp   ☐ Comfortable

Water

🥛 🥛 🥛 🥛 🥛 🥛 🥛 🥛

Energy Level

☆ ☆ ☆ ☆ ☆

Moon

- ☐ New Moon ●
- ☐ Waxing Crescent ●
- ☐ First Quarter ◐
- ☐ Waxing Gibbous ◑
- ☐ Full Moon ○
- ☐ Waning Gibbous ◔
- ☐ Third Quarter ◑
- ☐ Waning Crescent ◕

Bowel Movement

Constipation   *Diarrhea*

Type 1	Type 2	Type 3	Type 4	Type 5	Type 6	Type 7

Medications

Time	Description

Vitamins

Time	Description

Exercise

Time	Intensity	Activity

Breakfast

Lunch

Dinner

Snacks

Menstrual Cycle Symptoms

☐ Cramps ☐ Headache ☐ Backache ☐ Nausea ☐ Fatigue

☐ Tender Breasts ☐ Acne ☐ Bloating ☐ Cravings ☐ Insomnia

☐ Other

Physical Symptoms Log

Period

☐ Spotting ☐ Light ☐ Medium ☐ Heavy

Pain, Discomfort and Skin Changes

(See the Pain Level Reference and/or Glossary for help in describing your symptoms)

Describe your symptoms, pain level and approximate time in the appropriate space below:

☐ Head / Ears / Eyes / Nose / Mouth
_____
_____
_____

☐ Shoulders / Arms / Hands
_____
_____
_____

☐ Back
_____
_____
_____

☐ Lungs / Breathing (Respiratory)
_____
_____
_____

☐ Uterus / Vagina (Reproductive)
_____
_____
_____

☐ Other
_____
_____

☐ Throat / Neck
_____
_____
_____

☐ Chest / Heart
_____
_____
_____

☐ Hips / Buttocks / Legs / Feet
_____
_____
_____

☐ Stomach / Abdomen (Digestive)
_____
_____
_____

☐ Skin
_____
_____
_____

Mark all the places on the diagram below that you are experiencing pain, discomfort, and/or skin changes:

Front

Back

Notes
_____
_____
_____
_____
_____

Daily Wellness Log

Date: ....   S M T W Th F Sa

Weight:
Temperature:

Hours of Sleep

0 1 2 3 4 5 6 7 8 9 10 11 12+

Sleep Quality

☆ ☆ ☆ ☆ ☆

Weather

- [ ] Sunny ☀
- [ ] Partly Cloudy ☁
- [ ] Cloudy ⛅
- [ ] Windy 🌬
- [ ] Stormy ⛈
- [ ] Light Rain 🌧
- [ ] Heavy Rain 🌧
- [ ] Light Snow 🌨
- [ ] Heavy Snow 🌨
- [ ] Other ....

Mood

- [ ] Happy 🙂
- [ ] Calm 🙂
- [ ] Confident 😎
- [ ] Excited 😀
- [ ] Loving 😍
- [ ] Other ....
- [ ] Sad ☹
- [ ] Angry 😠
- [ ] Anxious 😧
- [ ] Stressed 😖
- [ ] Self-Critical 😠
- [ ] Tired 😣

Temperature

- [ ] Hot
- [ ] Warm
- [ ] Cold
- [ ] Damp
- [ ] Comfortable

Water

🥛 🥛 🥛 🥛 🥛 🥛 🥛 🥛

Energy Level

☆ ☆ ☆ ☆ ☆

Moon

- [ ] New Moon ●
- [ ] Waxing Crescent ●
- [ ] First Quarter ◑
- [ ] Waxing Gibbous ◑
- [ ] Full Moon ○
- [ ] Waning Gibbous ◐
- [ ] Third Quarter ◐
- [ ] Waning Crescent ◐

Bowel Movement

Constipation   *Diarrhea*

Type 1	Type 2	Type 3	Type 4	Type 5	Type 6	Type 7

Medications

Time	Description

Vitamins

Time	Description

Exercise

Time	Intensity	Activity

Breakfast

Lunch

Dinner

Snacks

Menstrual Cycle Symptoms

- [ ] Cramps
- [ ] Headache
- [ ] Backache
- [ ] Nausea
- [ ] Fatigue
- [ ] Tender Breasts
- [ ] Acne
- [ ] Bloating
- [ ] Cravings
- [ ] Insomnia
- [ ] Other

Physical Symptoms Log

Period

- [ ] Spotting
- [ ] Light
- [ ] Medium
- [ ] Heavy

Pain, Discomfort and Skin Changes

(See the Pain Level Reference and/or Glossary for help in describing your symptoms)

Describe your symptoms, pain level and approximate time in the appropriate space below:

- [ ] Head / Ears / Eyes / Nose / Mouth
_____
_____
_____

- [ ] Throat / Neck
_____
_____

- [ ] Shoulders / Arms / Hands
_____
_____
_____

- [ ] Chest / Heart
_____
_____
_____

- [ ] Back
_____
_____
_____

- [ ] Hips / Buttocks / Legs / Feet
_____
_____
_____

- [ ] Lungs / Breathing (Respiratory)
_____
_____

- [ ] Stomach / Abdomen (Digestive)
_____
_____

- [ ] Uterus / Vagina (Reproductive)
_____
_____

- [ ] Skin
_____
_____
_____

- [ ] Other
_____
_____

Mark all the places on the diagram below that you are experiencing pain, discomfort, and/or skin changes:

Front

Back

Notes
_____
_____
_____
_____

Daily Wellness Log

Date: ....   S M T W Th F Sa

Weight:
Temperature:

Hours of Sleep

0 1 2 3 4 5 6 7 8 9 10 11 12+

Sleep Quality

☆ ☆ ☆ ☆ ☆

Weather

- [ ] Sunny ☀
- [ ] Partly Cloudy ☁
- [ ] Cloudy ⛅
- [ ] Windy 🌬
- [ ] Stormy ⛈
- [ ] Light Rain 🌦
- [ ] Heavy Rain 🌧
- [ ] Light Snow 🌨
- [ ] Heavy Snow 🌨
- [ ] Other ....

Mood

- [ ] Happy ☺
- [ ] Calm ☺
- [ ] Confident 😎
- [ ] Excited 😄
- [ ] Loving 😍
- [ ] Other
- [ ] Sad ☹
- [ ] Angry 😠
- [ ] Anxious 😣
- [ ] Stressed 😫
- [ ] Self-Critical 😤
- [ ] Tired 😩

Temperature

- [ ] Hot
- [ ] Warm
- [ ] Cold
- [ ] Damp
- [ ] Comfortable

Water

🥛 🥛 🥛 🥛 🥛 🥛 🥛 🥛

Energy Level

☆ ☆ ☆ ☆ ☆

Moon

- [ ] New Moon ●
- [ ] Waxing Crescent ●
- [ ] First Quarter ◑
- [ ] Waxing Gibbous ◐
- [ ] Full Moon ○
- [ ] Waning Gibbous ◔
- [ ] Third Quarter ◐
- [ ] Waning Crescent ◖

Bowel Movement

Constipation   *Diarrhea*

Type 1   Type 2   Type 3   Type 4   Type 5   Type 6   Type 7

Medications

Time	Description

Vitamins

Time	Description

Exercise

Time	Intensity	Activity

Breakfast

Lunch

Dinner

Snacks

Menstrual Cycle Symptoms

☐ Cramps ☐ Headache ☐ Backache ☐ Nausea ☐ Fatigue

☐ Tender Breasts ☐ Acne ☐ Bloating ☐ Cravings ☐ Insomnia

☐ Other

Physical Symptoms Log

Period

☐ Spotting ☐ Light ☐ Medium ☐ Heavy

Pain, Discomfort and Skin Changes

(See the Pain Level Reference and/or Glossary for help in describing your symptoms)

Describe your symptoms, pain level and approximate time in the appropriate space below:

☐ Head / Ears / Eyes / Nose / Mouth
_____
_____
_____

☐ Shoulders / Arms / Hands
_____
_____
_____

☐ Back
_____
_____
_____

☐ Lungs / Breathing (Respiratory)
_____
_____
_____

☐ Uterus / Vagina (Reproductive)
_____
_____
_____

☐ Other
_____
_____

☐ Throat / Neck
_____
_____
_____

☐ Chest / Heart
_____
_____
_____

☐ Hips / Buttocks / Legs / Feet
_____
_____
_____

☐ Stomach / Abdomen (Digestive)
_____
_____
_____

☐ Skin
_____
_____
_____

Mark all the places on the diagram below that you are experiencing pain, discomfort, and/or skin changes:

Front

Back

Notes
_____
_____
_____
_____

Daily Wellness Log

Date: .... S M T W Th F Sa

Weight:
Temperature:

Hours of Sleep

0 1 2 3 4 5 6 7 8 9 10 11 12+

Sleep Quality

☆ ☆ ☆ ☆ ☆

Weather

- ☐ Sunny ☀
- ☐ Partly Cloudy ☁
- ☐ Cloudy ⛅
- ☐ Windy 🌬
- ☐ Stormy ⛈
- ☐ Light Rain 🌦
- ☐ Heavy Rain 🌧
- ☐ Light Snow 🌨
- ☐ Heavy Snow 🌨
- ☐ Other ....

Mood

- ☐ Happy ☺
- ☐ Calm ☺
- ☐ Confident 😎
- ☐ Excited 😄
- ☐ Loving 😍
- ☐ Other
- ☐ Sad ☹
- ☐ Angry 😠
- ☐ Anxious 😰
- ☐ Stressed 😖
- ☐ Self-Critical 😡
- ☐ Tired 😫

Temperature

☐ Hot ☐ Warm ☐ Cold ☐ Damp ☐ Comfortable

Water

🥛 🥛 🥛 🥛 🥛 🥛 🥛 🥛

Energy Level

☆ ☆ ☆ ☆ ☆

Moon

- ☐ New Moon ●
- ☐ Waxing Crescent ◗
- ☐ First Quarter ◑
- ☐ Waxing Gibbous ◐
- ☐ Full Moon ○
- ☐ Waning Gibbous ◖
- ☐ Third Quarter ◑
- ☐ Waning Crescent ◑

Bowel Movement

Constipation   *Diarrhea*

Type 1	Type 2	Type 3	Type 4	Type 5	Type 6	Type 7

Medications

Time	Description

Vitamins

Time	Description

Exercise

Time	Intensity	Activity

Breakfast

Lunch

Dinner

Snacks

Menstrual Cycle Symptoms

- [ ] Cramps
- [ ] Headache
- [ ] Backache
- [ ] Nausea
- [ ] Fatigue
- [ ] Tender Breasts
- [ ] Acne
- [ ] Bloating
- [ ] Cravings
- [ ] Insomnia
- [ ] Other

Physical Symptoms Log

Period

- [ ] Spotting
- [ ] Light
- [ ] Medium
- [ ] Heavy

Pain, Discomfort and Skin Changes

(See the Pain Level Reference and/or Glossary for help in describing your symptoms)

Describe your symptoms, pain level and approximate time in the appropriate space below:

- [ ] Head / Ears / Eyes / Nose / Mouth
- [ ] Throat / Neck
- [ ] Shoulders / Arms / Hands
- [ ] Chest / Heart
- [ ] Back
- [ ] Hips / Buttocks / Legs / Feet
- [ ] Lungs / Breathing (Respiratory)
- [ ] Stomach / Abdomen (Digestive)
- [ ] Uterus / Vagina (Reproductive)
- [ ] Skin
- [ ] Other

Mark all the places on the diagram below that you are experiencing pain, discomfort, and/or skin changes:

Front

Back

Notes

Daily Wellness Log

Date: .... S M T W Th F Sa

Weight: _____

Temperature: _____

Hours of Sleep

0 1 2 3 4 5 6 7 8 9 10 11 12+

Sleep Quality

☆ ☆ ☆ ☆ ☆

Weather

- ☐ Sunny ☀
- ☐ Partly Cloudy ☁
- ☐ Cloudy ⛅
- ☐ Windy 🌬
- ☐ Stormy ⛈
- ☐ Light Rain 🌦
- ☐ Heavy Rain 🌧
- ☐ Light Snow 🌨
- ☐ Heavy Snow 🌨
- ☐ Other ....

Mood

- ☐ Happy 🙂
- ☐ Calm 🙂
- ☐ Confident 😎
- ☐ Excited 😀
- ☐ Loving 😍
- ☐ Other
- ☐ Sad ☹
- ☐ Angry 😠
- ☐ Anxious 😟
- ☐ Stressed 😣
- ☐ Self-Critical 😤
- ☐ Tired 😫

Temperature

☐ Hot ☐ Warm ☐ Cold ☐ Damp ☐ Comfortable

Water

🥛 🥛 🥛 🥛 🥛 🥛 🥛 🥛

Energy Level

☆ ☆ ☆ ☆ ☆

Moon

- ☐ New Moon ●
- ☐ Waxing Crescent ◗
- ☐ First Quarter ◐
- ☐ Waxing Gibbous ◑
- ☐ Full Moon ○
- ☐ Waning Gibbous ◑
- ☐ Third Quarter ◐
- ☐ Waning Crescent ◗

Bowel Movement

Constipation   *Diarrhea*

Type 1   Type 2   Type 3   Type 4   Type 5   Type 6   Type 7

Medications

Time	Description

Vitamins

Time	Description

Exercise

Time	Intensity	Activity

Breakfast

Lunch

Dinner

Snacks

Menstrual Cycle Symptoms

- [ ] Cramps
- [ ] Headache
- [ ] Backache
- [ ] Nausea
- [ ] Fatigue
- [ ] Tender Breasts
- [ ] Acne
- [ ] Bloating
- [ ] Cravings
- [ ] Insomnia
- [ ] Other

Physical Symptoms Log

Period

- [ ] Spotting
- [ ] Light
- [ ] Medium
- [ ] Heavy

Pain, Discomfort and Skin Changes

(See the Pain Level Reference and/or Glossary for help in describing your symptoms)

Describe your symptoms, pain level and approximate time in the appropriate space below:

- [ ] Head / Ears / Eyes / Nose / Mouth
  _____
  _____
  _____

- [ ] Shoulders / Arms / Hands
  _____
  _____
  _____

- [ ] Back
  _____
  _____
  _____

- [ ] Lungs / Breathing (Respiratory)
  _____
  _____
  _____

- [ ] Uterus / Vagina (Reproductive)
  _____
  _____
  _____

- [ ] Other
  _____
  _____

- [ ] Throat / Neck
  _____
  _____
  _____

- [ ] Chest / Heart
  _____
  _____
  _____

- [ ] Hips / Buttocks / Legs / Feet
  _____
  _____
  _____

- [ ] Stomach / Abdomen (Digestive)
  _____
  _____
  _____

- [ ] Skin
  _____
  _____
  _____

Mark all the places on the diagram below that you are experiencing pain, discomfort, and/or skin changes:

Front

Back

Notes
_____
_____
_____
_____
_____

Daily Wellness Log

Date: ....   S M T W Th F Sa

Weight: _____
Temperature: _____

Hours of Sleep

0 1 2 3 4 5 6 7 8 9 10 11 12+

Sleep Quality

☆ ☆ ☆ ☆ ☆

Weather

- ☐ Sunny ☀
- ☐ Partly Cloudy ☁
- ☐ Cloudy ⛅
- ☐ Windy 🌬
- ☐ Stormy ⛈
- ☐ Light Rain 🌧
- ☐ Heavy Rain 🌧
- ☐ Light Snow 🌨
- ☐ Heavy Snow 🌨
- ☐ Other ....

Mood

- ☐ Happy 🙂
- ☐ Calm 🙂
- ☐ Confident 😎
- ☐ Excited 😃
- ☐ Loving 😍
- ☐ Other
- ☐ Sad 🙁
- ☐ Angry 😠
- ☐ Anxious 😟
- ☐ Stressed 😫
- ☐ Self-Critical 😠
- ☐ Tired 😩

Temperature

☐ Hot   ☐ Warm   ☐ Cold   ☐ Damp   ☐ Comfortable

Water

☐ ☐ ☐ ☐ ☐ ☐ ☐ ☐

Energy Level

☆ ☆ ☆ ☆ ☆

Moon

- ☐ New Moon ●
- ☐ Waxing Crescent ◐
- ☐ First Quarter ◑
- ☐ Waxing Gibbous ◑
- ☐ Full Moon ○
- ☐ Waning Gibbous ◑
- ☐ Third Quarter ◑
- ☐ Waning Crescent ◐

Bowel Movement

Constipation   *Diarrhea*

Type 1	Type 2	Type 3	Type 4	Type 5	Type 6	Type 7

Medications

Time	Description

Vitamins

Time	Description

Exercise

Time	Intensity	Activity

Breakfast

Lunch

Dinner

Snacks

Menstrual Cycle Symptoms

☐ Cramps ☐ Headache ☐ Backache ☐ Nausea ☐ Fatigue

☐ Tender Breasts ☐ Acne ☐ Bloating ☐ Cravings ☐ Insomnia

☐ Other

Physical Symptoms Log

Period

☐ Spotting ☐ Light ☐ Medium ☐ Heavy

Pain, Discomfort and Skin Changes

(See the Pain Level Reference and/or Glossary for help in describing your symptoms)

Describe your symptoms, pain level and approximate time in the appropriate space below:

☐ Head / Ears / Eyes / Nose / Mouth
_____
_____
_____

☐ Shoulders / Arms / Hands
_____
_____
_____

☐ Back
_____
_____
_____

☐ Lungs / Breathing (Respiratory)
_____
_____
_____

☐ Uterus / Vagina (Reproductive)
_____
_____
_____

☐ Other
_____
_____
_____

☐ Throat / Neck
_____
_____
_____

☐ Chest / Heart
_____
_____
_____

☐ Hips / Buttocks / Legs / Feet
_____
_____
_____

☐ Stomach / Abdomen (Digestive)
_____
_____
_____

☐ Skin
_____
_____
_____

Mark all the places on the diagram below that you are experiencing pain, discomfort, and/or skin changes:

Front

Back

Notes
_____
_____
_____
_____
_____

Daily Wellness Log

Date: ....   S M T W Th F Sa

Weight:

Temperature:

Hours of Sleep

0 1 2 3 4 5 6 7 8 9 10 11 12+

Sleep Quality

☆ ☆ ☆ ☆ ☆

Weather

- ☐ Sunny ☀
- ☐ Partly Cloudy ☁
- ☐ Cloudy ⛅
- ☐ Windy 🌬
- ☐ Stormy ⛈
- ☐ Light Rain 🌦
- ☐ Heavy Rain 🌧
- ☐ Light Snow 🌨
- ☐ Heavy Snow 🌨
- ☐ Other ....

Mood

- ☐ Happy ☺
- ☐ Calm ☺
- ☐ Confident 😎
- ☐ Excited ☺
- ☐ Loving 😍
- ☐ Other
- ☐ Sad ☹
- ☐ Angry 😠
- ☐ Anxious 😬
- ☐ Stressed 😖
- ☐ Self-Critical 😤
- ☐ Tired 😫

Temperature

☐ Hot   ☐ Warm   ☐ Cold   ☐ Damp   ☐ Comfortable

Water

🥛 🥛 🥛 🥛 🥛 🥛 🥛 🥛

Energy Level

☆ ☆ ☆ ☆ ☆

Moon

- ☐ New Moon ●
- ☐ Waxing Crescent ◗
- ☐ First Quarter ◐
- ☐ Waxing Gibbous ◑
- ☐ Full Moon ○
- ☐ Waning Gibbous ◔
- ☐ Third Quarter ◑
- ☐ Waning Crescent ◕

Bowel Movement

Constipation   *Diarrhea*

Type 1	Type 2	Type 3	Type 4	Type 5	Type 6	Type 7

Medications

Time	Description

Vitamins

Time	Description

Exercise

Time	Intensity	Activity

Breakfast

Lunch

Dinner

Snacks

Menstrual Cycle Symptoms

- [ ] Cramps
- [ ] Headache
- [ ] Backache
- [ ] Nausea
- [ ] Fatigue
- [ ] Tender Breasts
- [ ] Acne
- [ ] Bloating
- [ ] Cravings
- [ ] Insomnia
- [ ] Other

Physical Symptoms Log

Period

- [ ] Spotting
- [ ] Light
- [ ] Medium
- [ ] Heavy

Pain, Discomfort and Skin Changes

(See the Pain Level Reference and/or Glossary for help in describing your symptoms)

Describe your symptoms, pain level and approximate time in the appropriate space below:

- [ ] Head / Ears / Eyes / Nose / Mouth

- [ ] Throat / Neck

- [ ] Shoulders / Arms / Hands

- [ ] Chest / Heart

- [ ] Back

- [ ] Hips / Buttocks / Legs / Feet

- [ ] Lungs / Breathing (Respiratory)

- [ ] Stomach / Abdomen (Digestive)

- [ ] Uterus / Vagina (Reproductive)

- [ ] Skin

- [ ] Other

Mark all the places on the diagram below that you are experiencing pain, discomfort, and/or skin changes:

Front

Back

Notes

Daily Wellness Log

Date: ....   S M T W Th F Sa

Weight: _____

Temperature: _____

Hours of Sleep

0 1 2 3 4 5 6 7 8 9 10 11 12+

Sleep Quality

☆ ☆ ☆ ☆ ☆

Weather

- [ ] Sunny ☼
- [ ] Partly Cloudy
- [ ] Cloudy
- [ ] Windy
- [ ] Stormy
- [ ] Light Rain
- [ ] Heavy Rain
- [ ] Light Snow
- [ ] Heavy Snow
- [ ] Other ....

Mood

- [ ] Happy ☺
- [ ] Calm ☺
- [ ] Confident 😎
- [ ] Excited ☺
- [ ] Loving 😍
- [ ] Other
- [ ] Sad ☹
- [ ] Angry 😠
- [ ] Anxious 😣
- [ ] Stressed 😣
- [ ] Self-Critical 😠
- [ ] Tired 😫

Temperature

- [ ] Hot
- [ ] Warm
- [ ] Cold
- [ ] Damp
- [ ] Comfortable

Water

▽ ▽ ▽ ▽ ▽ ▽ ▽ ▽

Energy Level

☆ ☆ ☆ ☆ ☆

Moon

- [ ] New Moon ●
- [ ] Waxing Crescent ●
- [ ] First Quarter ◐
- [ ] Waxing Gibbous ◐
- [ ] Full Moon ○
- [ ] Waning Gibbous ◐
- [ ] Third Quarter ◐
- [ ] Waning Crescent ●

Bowel Movement

Constipation   *Diarrhea*

Type 1	Type 2	Type 3	Type 4	Type 5	Type 6	Type 7

Medications

Time	Description

Vitamins

Time	Description

Exercise

Time	Intensity	Activity

Breakfast

Lunch

Dinner

Snacks

Menstrual Cycle Symptoms

- [ ] Cramps
- [ ] Headache
- [ ] Backache
- [ ] Nausea
- [ ] Fatigue
- [ ] Tender Breasts
- [ ] Acne
- [ ] Bloating
- [ ] Cravings
- [ ] Insomnia
- [ ] Other

Physical Symptoms Log

Period

- [ ] Spotting
- [ ] Light
- [ ] Medium
- [ ] Heavy

Pain, Discomfort and Skin Changes

(See the Pain Level Reference and/or Glossary for help in describing your symptoms)

Describe your symptoms, pain level and approximate time in the appropriate space below:

- [ ] Head / Ears / Eyes / Nose / Mouth
- [ ] Throat / Neck
- [ ] Shoulders / Arms / Hands
- [ ] Chest / Heart
- [ ] Back
- [ ] Hips / Buttocks / Legs / Feet
- [ ] Lungs / Breathing (Respiratory)
- [ ] Stomach / Abdomen (Digestive)
- [ ] Uterus / Vagina (Reproductive)
- [ ] Skin
- [ ] Other

Mark all the places on the diagram below that you are experiencing pain, discomfort, and/or skin changes:

Front

Back

Notes

Daily Wellness Log

Date: ....   S M T W Th F Sa

Weight: _____
Temperature: _____

Hours of Sleep

0   1   2   3   4   5   6   7   8   9   10   11   12+

Sleep Quality

☆ ☆ ☆ ☆ ☆

Weather

- [ ] Sunny ☀
- [ ] Partly Cloudy ☁
- [ ] Cloudy ⛅
- [ ] Windy 🌬
- [ ] Stormy ⛈
- [ ] Light Rain 🌦
- [ ] Heavy Rain 🌧
- [ ] Light Snow 🌨
- [ ] Heavy Snow 🌨
- [ ] Other ....

Mood

- [ ] Happy 🙂
- [ ] Calm 🙂
- [ ] Confident 😎
- [ ] Excited 😄
- [ ] Loving 😍
- [ ] Other
- [ ] Sad 🙁
- [ ] Angry 😠
- [ ] Anxious 😟
- [ ] Stressed 😣
- [ ] Self-Critical 😈
- [ ] Tired 😫

Temperature

- [ ] Hot
- [ ] Warm
- [ ] Cold
- [ ] Damp
- [ ] Comfortable

Water

🥛 🥛 🥛 🥛 🥛 🥛 🥛 🥛

Energy Level

☆ ☆ ☆ ☆ ☆

Moon

- [ ] New Moon ●
- [ ] Waxing Crescent ●
- [ ] First Quarter ◐
- [ ] Waxing Gibbous ◑
- [ ] Full Moon ○
- [ ] Waning Gibbous ○
- [ ] Third Quarter ◑
- [ ] Waning Crescent ◐

Bowel Movement

Constipation   *Diarrhea*

Type 1   Type 2   Type 3   Type 4   Type 5   Type 6   Type 7

Medications

Time	Description

Vitamins

Time	Description

Exercise

Time	Intensity	Activity

Breakfast

Lunch

Dinner

Snacks

Menstrual Cycle Symptoms

- [ ] Cramps
- [ ] Headache
- [ ] Backache
- [ ] Nausea
- [ ] Fatigue
- [ ] Tender Breasts
- [ ] Acne
- [ ] Bloating
- [ ] Cravings
- [ ] Insomnia
- [ ] Other

Physical Symptoms Log

Period

- [ ] Spotting
- [ ] Light
- [ ] Medium
- [ ] Heavy

Pain, Discomfort and Skin Changes

(See the Pain Level Reference and/or Glossary for help in describing your symptoms)

Describe your symptoms, pain level and approximate time in the appropriate space below:

- [ ] Head / Ears / Eyes / Nose / Mouth
- [ ] Throat / Neck
- [ ] Shoulders / Arms / Hands
- [ ] Chest / Heart
- [ ] Back
- [ ] Hips / Buttocks / Legs / Feet
- [ ] Lungs / Breathing (Respiratory)
- [ ] Stomach / Abdomen (Digestive)
- [ ] Uterus / Vagina (Reproductive)
- [ ] Skin
- [ ] Other

Mark all the places on the diagram below that you are experiencing pain, discomfort, and/or skin changes:

Front

Back

Notes

Daily Wellness Log

Date: ....   S M T W Th F Sa

Weight:
Temperature:

Hours of Sleep
0 1 2 3 4 5 6 7 8 9 10 11 12+

Sleep Quality
☆ ☆ ☆ ☆ ☆

Weather
- [ ] Sunny ☀
- [ ] Partly Cloudy ☁
- [ ] Cloudy ⛅
- [ ] Windy 🌬
- [ ] Stormy ⛈
- [ ] Light Rain 🌧
- [ ] Heavy Rain 🌧
- [ ] Light Snow 🌨
- [ ] Heavy Snow 🌨
- [ ] Other ....

Mood
- [ ] Happy ☺
- [ ] Calm ☺
- [ ] Confident 😎
- [ ] Excited ☺
- [ ] Loving 😍
- [ ] Other
- [ ] Sad ☹
- [ ] Angry 😠
- [ ] Anxious 😟
- [ ] Stressed 😣
- [ ] Self-Critical 😡
- [ ] Tired 😫

Temperature
- [ ] Hot
- [ ] Warm
- [ ] Cold
- [ ] Damp
- [ ] Comfortable

Water
🥛 🥛 🥛 🥛 🥛 🥛 🥛 🥛

Energy Level
☆ ☆ ☆ ☆ ☆

Moon
- [ ] New Moon ●
- [ ] Waxing Crescent ◐
- [ ] First Quarter ◑
- [ ] Waxing Gibbous ◑
- [ ] Full Moon ○
- [ ] Waning Gibbous ◔
- [ ] Third Quarter ◑
- [ ] Waning Crescent ◐

Bowel Movement
Constipation   *Diarrhea*

Type 1	Type 2	Type 3	Type 4	Type 5	Type 6	Type 7

Medications

Time	Description

Vitamins

Time	Description

Exercise

Time	Intensity	Activity

Breakfast

Lunch

Dinner

Snacks

Menstrual Cycle Symptoms

- [ ] Cramps
- [ ] Headache
- [ ] Backache
- [ ] Nausea
- [ ] Fatigue
- [ ] Tender Breasts
- [ ] Acne
- [ ] Bloating
- [ ] Cravings
- [ ] Insomnia
- [ ] Other

Physical Symptoms Log

Period

- [ ] Spotting
- [ ] Light
- [ ] Medium
- [ ] Heavy

Pain, Discomfort and Skin Changes

(See the Pain Level Reference and/or Glossary for help in describing your symptoms)

Describe your symptoms, pain level and approximate time in the appropriate space below:

- [ ] Head / Ears / Eyes / Nose / Mouth
- [ ] Throat / Neck
- [ ] Shoulders / Arms / Hands
- [ ] Chest / Heart
- [ ] Back
- [ ] Hips / Buttocks / Legs / Feet
- [ ] Lungs / Breathing (Respiratory)
- [ ] Stomach / Abdomen (Digestive)
- [ ] Uterus / Vagina (Reproductive)
- [ ] Skin
- [ ] Other

Mark all the places on the diagram below that you are experiencing pain, discomfort, and/or skin changes:

Front

Back

Notes

Daily Wellness Log

Date: _____   S M T W Th F Sa

Weight: _____
Temperature: _____

Hours of Sleep

0 1 2 3 4 5 6 7 8 9 10 11 12+

Sleep Quality

☆ ☆ ☆ ☆ ☆

Weather

- [ ] Sunny ☀
- [ ] Partly Cloudy ☁
- [ ] Cloudy ⛅
- [ ] Windy 🌬
- [ ] Stormy ⛈
- [ ] Light Rain 🌦
- [ ] Heavy Rain 🌧
- [ ] Light Snow 🌨
- [ ] Heavy Snow 🌨
- [ ] Other ....

Mood

- [ ] Happy ☺
- [ ] Calm ☺
- [ ] Confident 😎
- [ ] Excited 😄
- [ ] Loving 😍
- [ ] Other
- [ ] Sad ☹
- [ ] Angry 😠
- [ ] Anxious 😟
- [ ] Stressed 😣
- [ ] Self-Critical 😤
- [ ] Tired 😫

Temperature

- [ ] Hot
- [ ] Warm
- [ ] Cold
- [ ] Damp
- [ ] Comfortable

Water

🥤 🥤 🥤 🥤 🥤 🥤 🥤 🥤

Energy Level

☆ ☆ ☆ ☆ ☆

Moon

- [ ] New Moon ●
- [ ] Waxing Crescent ◐
- [ ] First Quarter ◑
- [ ] Waxing Gibbous ◑
- [ ] Full Moon ○
- [ ] Waning Gibbous ◑
- [ ] Third Quarter ◑
- [ ] Waning Crescent ◐

Bowel Movement

Constipation   *Diarrhea*

Type 1	Type 2	Type 3	Type 4	Type 5	Type 6	Type 7

Medications

Time	Description

Vitamins

Time	Description

Exercise

Time	Intensity	Activity

Breakfast

Lunch

Dinner

Snacks

Menstrual Cycle Symptoms

- [ ] Cramps
- [ ] Headache
- [ ] Backache
- [ ] Nausea
- [ ] Fatigue
- [ ] Tender Breasts
- [ ] Acne
- [ ] Bloating
- [ ] Cravings
- [ ] Insomnia
- [ ] Other

Physical Symptoms Log

Period

- [ ] Spotting
- [ ] Light
- [ ] Medium
- [ ] Heavy

Pain, Discomfort and Skin Changes

(See the Pain Level Reference and/or Glossary for help in describing your symptoms)

Describe your symptoms, pain level and approximate time in the appropriate space below:

- [ ] Head / Ears / Eyes / Nose / Mouth
- [ ] Throat / Neck
- [ ] Shoulders / Arms / Hands
- [ ] Chest / Heart
- [ ] Back
- [ ] Hips / Buttocks / Legs / Feet
- [ ] Lungs / Breathing (Respiratory)
- [ ] Stomach / Abdomen (Digestive)
- [ ] Uterus / Vagina (Reproductive)
- [ ] Skin
- [ ] Other

Mark all the places on the diagram below that you are experiencing pain, discomfort, and/or skin changes:

Front

Back

Notes

Daily Wellness Log

Date: ....   S M T W Th F Sa

Weight:
Temperature:

Hours of Sleep

0 1 2 3 4 5 6 7 8 9 10 11 12+

Sleep Quality

☆ ☆ ☆ ☆ ☆

Weather

- ☐ Sunny ☀
- ☐ Partly Cloudy ☁
- ☐ Cloudy ⛅
- ☐ Windy 🌬
- ☐ Stormy ⛈
- ☐ Light Rain 🌦
- ☐ Heavy Rain 🌧
- ☐ Light Snow 🌨
- ☐ Heavy Snow 🌨
- ☐ Other ....

Mood

- ☐ Happy
- ☐ Calm
- ☐ Confident
- ☐ Excited
- ☐ Loving
- ☐ Other
- ☐ Sad
- ☐ Angry
- ☐ Anxious
- ☐ Stressed
- ☐ Self-Critical
- ☐ Tired

Temperature

☐ Hot ☐ Warm ☐ Cold ☐ Damp ☐ Comfortable

Water

☐ ☐ ☐ ☐ ☐ ☐ ☐ ☐

Energy Level

☆ ☆ ☆ ☆ ☆

Moon

- ☐ New Moon
- ☐ Waxing Crescent
- ☐ First Quarter
- ☐ Waxing Gibbous
- ☐ Full Moon
- ☐ Waning Gibbous
- ☐ Third Quarter
- ☐ Waning Crescent

Bowel Movement

Constipation .... *Diarrhea*

Type 1	Type 2	Type 3	Type 4	Type 5	Type 6	Type 7

Medications

Time	Description

Vitamins

Time	Description

Exercise

Time	Intensity	Activity

Breakfast

Lunch

Dinner

Snacks

Menstrual Cycle Symptoms

- [ ] Cramps
- [ ] Headache
- [ ] Backache
- [ ] Nausea
- [ ] Fatigue
- [ ] Tender Breasts
- [ ] Acne
- [ ] Bloating
- [ ] Cravings
- [ ] Insomnia
- [ ] Other

Physical Symptoms Log

Period

- [ ] Spotting
- [ ] Light
- [ ] Medium
- [ ] Heavy

Pain, Discomfort and Skin Changes

(See the Pain Level Reference and/or Glossary for help in describing your symptoms)

Describe your symptoms, pain level and approximate time in the appropriate space below:

- [ ] Head / Ears / Eyes / Nose / Mouth

- [ ] Throat / Neck

- [ ] Shoulders / Arms / Hands

- [ ] Chest / Heart

- [ ] Back

- [ ] Hips / Buttocks / Legs / Feet

- [ ] Lungs / Breathing (Respiratory)

- [ ] Stomach / Abdomen (Digestive)

- [ ] Uterus / Vagina (Reproductive)

- [ ] Skin

- [ ] Other

Mark all the places on the diagram below that you are experiencing pain, discomfort, and/or skin changes:

Front

Back

Notes

Daily Wellness Log

Date: ....   S M T W Th F Sa

Weight:
Temperature:

Hours of Sleep

0 1 2 3 4 5 6 7 8 9 10 11 12+

Sleep Quality
☆ ☆ ☆ ☆ ☆

Weather

- [ ] Sunny ☀
- [ ] Partly Cloudy ☁
- [ ] Cloudy ⛅
- [ ] Windy 🌬
- [ ] Stormy ⛈

- [ ] Light Rain 🌦
- [ ] Heavy Rain 🌧
- [ ] Light Snow 🌨
- [ ] Heavy Snow 🌨
- [ ] Other ....

Mood

- [ ] Happy 🙂
- [ ] Calm 🙂
- [ ] Confident 😎
- [ ] Excited 😃
- [ ] Loving 😍
- [ ] Other

- [ ] Sad ☹
- [ ] Angry 😠
- [ ] Anxious 😣
- [ ] Stressed 😖
- [ ] Self-Critical 😤
- [ ] Tired 😫

Temperature

- [ ] Hot
- [ ] Warm
- [ ] Cold
- [ ] Damp
- [ ] Comfortable

Water

🥛 🥛 🥛 🥛 🥛 🥛 🥛 🥛

Energy Level
☆ ☆ ☆ ☆ ☆

Moon

- [ ] New Moon ●
- [ ] Waxing Crescent ◗
- [ ] First Quarter ◐
- [ ] Waxing Gibbous ◑

- [ ] Full Moon ○
- [ ] Waning Gibbous ◔
- [ ] Third Quarter ◑
- [ ] Waning Crescent ◕

Bowel Movement

Constipation   *Diarrhea*

Type 1	Type 2	Type 3	Type 4	Type 5	Type 6	Type 7

Medications

Time	Description

Vitamins

Time	Description

Exercise

Time	Intensity	Activity

Breakfast

Lunch

Dinner

Snacks

Menstrual Cycle Symptoms

- [ ] Cramps
- [ ] Headache
- [ ] Backache
- [ ] Nausea
- [ ] Fatigue
- [ ] Tender Breasts
- [ ] Acne
- [ ] Bloating
- [ ] Cravings
- [ ] Insomnia
- [ ] Other

Physical Symptoms Log

Period

- [ ] Spotting
- [ ] Light
- [ ] Medium
- [ ] Heavy

Pain, Discomfort and Skin Changes

(See the Pain Level Reference and/or Glossary for help in describing your symptoms)

Describe your symptoms, pain level and approximate time in the appropriate space below:

- [ ] Head / Ears / Eyes / Nose / Mouth
- [ ] Throat / Neck

- [ ] Shoulders / Arms / Hands
- [ ] Chest / Heart

- [ ] Back
- [ ] Hips / Buttocks / Legs / Feet

- [ ] Lungs / Breathing (Respiratory)
- [ ] Stomach / Abdomen (Digestive)

- [ ] Uterus / Vagina (Reproductive)
- [ ] Skin

- [ ] Other

Mark all the places on the diagram below that you are experiencing pain, discomfort, and/or skin changes:

Front

Back

Notes

Daily Wellness Log

Date: ....   S M T W Th F Sa

Weight:

Temperature:

Hours of Sleep

0 1 2 3 4 5 6 7 8 9 10 11 12+

Sleep Quality

☆ ☆ ☆ ☆ ☆

Weather

- ☐ Sunny
- ☐ Partly Cloudy
- ☐ Cloudy
- ☐ Windy
- ☐ Stormy
- ☐ Light Rain
- ☐ Heavy Rain
- ☐ Light Snow
- ☐ Heavy Snow
- ☐ Other ....

Mood

- ☐ Happy
- ☐ Calm
- ☐ Confident
- ☐ Excited
- ☐ Loving
- ☐ Other
- ☐ Sad
- ☐ Angry
- ☐ Anxious
- ☐ Stressed
- ☐ Self-Critical
- ☐ Tired

Temperature

☐ Hot   ☐ Warm   ☐ Cold   ☐ Damp   ☐ Comfortable

Water

☐ ☐ ☐ ☐ ☐ ☐ ☐ ☐

Energy Level

☆ ☆ ☆ ☆ ☆

Moon

- ☐ New Moon
- ☐ Waxing Crescent
- ☐ First Quarter
- ☐ Waxing Gibbous
- ☐ Full Moon
- ☐ Waning Gibbous
- ☐ Third Quarter
- ☐ Waning Crescent

Bowel Movement

Constipation   *Diarrhea*

Type 1	Type 2	Type 3	Type 4	Type 5	Type 6	Type 7

Medications

Time	Description

Vitamins

Time	Description

Exercise

Time	Intensity	Activity

Breakfast

Lunch

Dinner

Snacks

Menstrual Cycle Symptoms

☐ Cramps ☐ Headache ☐ Backache ☐ Nausea ☐ Fatigue

☐ Tender Breasts ☐ Acne ☐ Bloating ☐ Cravings ☐ Insomnia

☐ Other

Physical Symptoms Log

Period

☐ Spotting ☐ Light ☐ Medium ☐ Heavy

Pain, Discomfort and Skin Changes

(See the Pain Level Reference and/or Glossary for help in describing your symptoms)

Describe your symptoms, pain level and approximate time in the appropriate space below:

☐ Head / Ears / Eyes / Nose / Mouth

_____
_____
_____

☐ Shoulders / Arms / Hands

_____
_____
_____

☐ Back

_____
_____
_____

☐ Lungs / Breathing (Respiratory)

_____
_____
_____

☐ Uterus / Vagina (Reproductive)

_____
_____
_____

☐ Other

_____
_____
_____

☐ Throat / Neck

_____
_____
_____

☐ Chest / Heart

_____
_____
_____

☐ Hips / Buttocks / Legs / Feet

_____
_____
_____

☐ Stomach / Abdomen (Digestive)

_____
_____
_____

☐ Skin

_____
_____
_____

Mark all the places on the diagram below that you are experiencing pain, discomfort, and/or skin changes:

Front

Back

Notes

Daily Wellness Log

Date: ....   S M T W Th F Sa

Weight: ....
Temperature: ....

Hours of Sleep

0 1 2 3 4 5 6 7 8 9 10 11 12+

Sleep Quality

☆ ☆ ☆ ☆ ☆

Weather

- [ ] Sunny ☀
- [ ] Partly Cloudy ☁
- [ ] Cloudy ⛅
- [ ] Windy 🌬
- [ ] Stormy ⛈
- [ ] Light Rain 🌦
- [ ] Heavy Rain 🌧
- [ ] Light Snow 🌨
- [ ] Heavy Snow 🌨
- [ ] Other ....

Mood

- [ ] Happy 🙂
- [ ] Calm 🙂
- [ ] Confident 😎
- [ ] Excited 😀
- [ ] Loving 😍
- [ ] Other ....
- [ ] Sad 🙁
- [ ] Angry 😠
- [ ] Anxious 😟
- [ ] Stressed 😣
- [ ] Self-Critical 😈
- [ ] Tired 😫

Temperature

- [ ] Hot
- [ ] Warm
- [ ] Cold
- [ ] Damp
- [ ] Comfortable

Water

🥛 🥛 🥛 🥛 🥛 🥛 🥛 🥛

Energy Level

☆ ☆ ☆ ☆ ☆

Moon

- [ ] New Moon ●
- [ ] Waxing Crescent ●
- [ ] First Quarter ◐
- [ ] Waxing Gibbous ◐
- [ ] Full Moon ○
- [ ] Waning Gibbous ◑
- [ ] Third Quarter ◑
- [ ] Waning Crescent ◑

Bowel Movement

Constipation   Diarrhea

Type 1	Type 2	Type 3	Type 4	Type 5	Type 6	Type 7

Medications

Time	Description

Vitamins

Time	Description

Exercise

Time	Intensity	Activity

Breakfast

Lunch

Dinner

Snacks

Menstrual Cycle Symptoms

- [ ] Cramps
- [ ] Headache
- [ ] Backache
- [ ] Nausea
- [ ] Fatigue
- [ ] Tender Breasts
- [ ] Acne
- [ ] Bloating
- [ ] Cravings
- [ ] Insomnia
- [ ] Other _____

Physical Symptoms Log

Period

- [ ] Spotting
- [ ] Light
- [ ] Medium
- [ ] Heavy

Pain, Discomfort and Skin Changes

(See the Pain Level Reference and/or Glossary for help in describing your symptoms)

Describe your symptoms, pain level and approximate time in the appropriate space below:

- [ ] Head / Ears / Eyes / Nose / Mouth
  _____
  _____
  _____

- [ ] Throat / Neck
  _____
  _____

- [ ] Shoulders / Arms / Hands
  _____
  _____
  _____

- [ ] Chest / Heart
  _____
  _____

- [ ] Back
  _____
  _____
  _____

- [ ] Hips / Buttocks / Legs / Feet
  _____
  _____

- [ ] Lungs / Breathing (Respiratory)
  _____
  _____

- [ ] Stomach / Abdomen (Digestive)
  _____
  _____

- [ ] Uterus / Vagina (Reproductive)
  _____
  _____
  _____

- [ ] Skin
  _____
  _____

- [ ] Other
  _____
  _____

Mark all the places on the diagram below that you are experiencing pain, discomfort, and/or skin changes:

Front

Back

Notes

_____
_____
_____
_____

Daily Wellness Log

Date: _____   S M T W Th F Sa

Weight: _____
Temperature: _____

Hours of Sleep

0 1 2 3 4 5 6 7 8 9 10 11 12+

Sleep Quality

☆ ☆ ☆ ☆ ☆

Weather

- [ ] Sunny ☀
- [ ] Partly Cloudy ☁
- [ ] Cloudy ⛅
- [ ] Windy 🌬
- [ ] Stormy ⛈
- [ ] Light Rain 🌦
- [ ] Heavy Rain 🌧
- [ ] Light Snow 🌨
- [ ] Heavy Snow 🌨
- [ ] Other

Mood

- [ ] Happy ☺
- [ ] Calm ☺
- [ ] Confident 😎
- [ ] Excited ☺
- [ ] Loving 😍
- [ ] Other
- [ ] Sad ☹
- [ ] Angry 😠
- [ ] Anxious 😣
- [ ] Stressed 😫
- [ ] Self-Critical 😡
- [ ] Tired 😫

Temperature

- [ ] Hot
- [ ] Warm
- [ ] Cold
- [ ] Damp
- [ ] Comfortable

Water

[ ] [ ] [ ] [ ] [ ] [ ] [ ] [ ]

Energy Level

☆ ☆ ☆ ☆ ☆

Moon

- [ ] New Moon ●
- [ ] Waxing Crescent ●
- [ ] First Quarter ◑
- [ ] Waxing Gibbous ◑
- [ ] Full Moon ○
- [ ] Waning Gibbous ◐
- [ ] Third Quarter ◐
- [ ] Waning Crescent ◐

Bowel Movement

Constipation   *Diarrhea*

Type 1   Type 2   Type 3   Type 4   Type 5   Type 6   Type 7

Medications

Time	Description

Vitamins

Time	Description

Exercise

Time	Intensity	Activity

Breakfast

Lunch

Dinner

Snacks

Menstrual Cycle Symptoms

- [ ] Cramps
- [ ] Headache
- [ ] Backache
- [ ] Nausea
- [ ] Fatigue
- [ ] Tender Breasts
- [ ] Acne
- [ ] Bloating
- [ ] Cravings
- [ ] Insomnia
- [ ] Other

Physical Symptoms Log

Period

- [ ] Spotting
- [ ] Light
- [ ] Medium
- [ ] Heavy

Pain, Discomfort and Skin Changes

(See the Pain Level Reference and/or Glossary for help in describing your symptoms)

Describe your symptoms, pain level and approximate time in the appropriate space below:

- [ ] Head / Ears / Eyes / Nose / Mouth

- [ ] Throat / Neck

- [ ] Shoulders / Arms / Hands

- [ ] Chest / Heart

- [ ] Back

- [ ] Hips / Buttocks / Legs / Feet

- [ ] Lungs / Breathing (Respiratory)

- [ ] Stomach / Abdomen (Digestive)

- [ ] Uterus / Vagina (Reproductive)

- [ ] Skin

- [ ] Other

Mark all the places on the diagram below that you are experiencing pain, discomfort, and/or skin changes:

Front

Back

Notes

Daily Wellness Log

Date: .... S M T W Th F Sa

Weight: ....
Temperature: ....

Hours of Sleep

0 1 2 3 4 5 6 7 8 9 10 11 12+

Sleep Quality

☆ ☆ ☆ ☆ ☆

Weather

- [ ] Sunny ☀
- [ ] Partly Cloudy ☁
- [ ] Cloudy ⛅
- [ ] Windy 🌬
- [ ] Stormy ⛈
- [ ] Light Rain 🌦
- [ ] Heavy Rain 🌧
- [ ] Light Snow 🌨
- [ ] Heavy Snow 🌨
- [ ] Other ....

Mood

- [ ] Happy 🙂
- [ ] Calm 🙂
- [ ] Confident 😎
- [ ] Excited 😀
- [ ] Loving 😍
- [ ] Other
- [ ] Sad ☹
- [ ] Angry 😠
- [ ] Anxious 😟
- [ ] Stressed 😣
- [ ] Self-Critical 😤
- [ ] Tired 😫

Temperature

- [ ] Hot
- [ ] Warm
- [ ] Cold
- [ ] Damp
- [ ] Comfortable

Water

🥤 🥤 🥤 🥤 🥤 🥤 🥤 🥤

Energy Level

☆ ☆ ☆ ☆ ☆

Moon

- [ ] New Moon ●
- [ ] Waxing Crescent ●
- [ ] First Quarter ◐
- [ ] Waxing Gibbous ◑
- [ ] Full Moon ○
- [ ] Waning Gibbous ◑
- [ ] Third Quarter ◐
- [ ] Waning Crescent ◐

Bowel Movement

Constipation   Diarrhea

Type 1   Type 2   Type 3   Type 4   Type 5   Type 6   Type 7

Medication

Time	Description

Vitamins

Time	Description

Exercise

Time	Intensity	Activity

Breakfast

Lunch

Dinner

Snacks

Menstrual Cycle Symptoms

- [ ] Cramps
- [ ] Headache
- [ ] Backache
- [ ] Nausea
- [ ] Fatigue
- [ ] Tender Breasts
- [ ] Acne
- [ ] Bloating
- [ ] Cravings
- [ ] Insomnia
- [ ] Other

Physical Symptoms Log

Period

- [ ] Spotting
- [ ] Light
- [ ] Medium
- [ ] Heavy

Pain, Discomfort and Skin Changes

(See the Pain Level Reference and/or Glossary for help in describing your symptoms)

Describe your symptoms, pain level and approximate time in the appropriate space below:

- [ ] Head / Ears / Eyes / Nose / Mouth

- [ ] Throat / Neck

- [ ] Shoulders / Arms / Hands

- [ ] Chest / Heart

- [ ] Back

- [ ] Hips / Buttocks / Legs / Feet

- [ ] Lungs / Breathing (Respiratory)

- [ ] Stomach / Abdomen (Digestive)

- [ ] Uterus / Vagina (Reproductive)

- [ ] Skin

- [ ] Other

Mark all the places on the diagram below that you are experiencing pain, discomfort, and/or skin changes:

Front

Back

Notes

Daily Wellness Log

Date: ....   S M T W Th F Sa

Weight: ....
Temperature: ....

Hours of Sleep

0 1 2 3 4 5 6 7 8 9 10 11 12+

Sleep Quality

☆ ☆ ☆ ☆ ☆

Weather

- [ ] Sunny ☀
- [ ] Partly Cloudy ☁
- [ ] Cloudy ⛅
- [ ] Windy 🌬
- [ ] Stormy ⛈
- [ ] Light Rain 🌦
- [ ] Heavy Rain 🌧
- [ ] Light Snow 🌨
- [ ] Heavy Snow 🌨
- [ ] Other ....

Mood

- [ ] Happy 🙂
- [ ] Calm 🙂
- [ ] Confident 😎
- [ ] Excited 😀
- [ ] Loving 😍
- [ ] Other
- [ ] Sad ☹
- [ ] Angry 😠
- [ ] Anxious 😧
- [ ] Stressed 😖
- [ ] Self-Critical 😡
- [ ] Tired 😫

Temperature

- [ ] Hot
- [ ] Warm
- [ ] Cold
- [ ] Damp
- [ ] Comfortable

Water

🥛 🥛 🥛 🥛 🥛 🥛 🥛 🥛

Energy Level

☆ ☆ ☆ ☆ ☆

Moon

- [ ] New Moon ●
- [ ] Waxing Crescent ●
- [ ] First Quarter ◑
- [ ] Waxing Gibbous ◗
- [ ] Full Moon ○
- [ ] Waning Gibbous ◐
- [ ] Third Quarter ◐
- [ ] Waning Crescent ◖

Bowel Movement

Constipation   *Diarrhea*

Type 1	Type 2	Type 3	Type 4	Type 5	Type 6	Type 7

Medication

Time	Description

Vitamins

Time	Description

Exercise

Time	Intensity	Activity

Breakfast

Lunch

Dinner

Snacks

Menstrual Cycle Symptoms

☐ Cramps ☐ Headache ☐ Backache ☐ Nausea ☐ Fatigue

☐ Tender Breasts ☐ Acne ☐ Bloating ☐ Cravings ☐ Insomnia

☐ Other

Physical Symptoms Log

Period

☐ Spotting ☐ Light ☐ Medium ☐ Heavy

Pain, Discomfort and Skin Changes

(See the Pain Level Reference and/or Glossary for help in describing your symptoms)

Describe your symptoms, pain level and approximate time in the appropriate space below:

☐ Head / Ears / Eyes / Nose / Mouth

_____
_____
_____

☐ Shoulders / Arms / Hands

_____
_____
_____

☐ Back

_____
_____
_____

☐ Lungs / Breathing (Respiratory)

_____
_____
_____

☐ Uterus / Vagina (Reproductive)

_____
_____
_____

☐ Other

_____
_____

☐ Throat / Neck

_____
_____
_____

☐ Chest / Heart

_____
_____
_____

☐ Hips / Buttocks / Legs / Feet

_____
_____
_____

☐ Stomach / Abdomen (Digestive)

_____
_____
_____

☐ Skin

_____
_____
_____

Mark all the places on the diagram below that you are experiencing pain, discomfort, and/or skin changes:

Front

Back

Notes

_____
_____
_____
_____

Daily Wellness Log

Date: ....   S M T W Th F Sa

Weight:
Temperature:

Hours of Sleep

0 1 2 3 4 5 6 7 8 9 10 11 12+

Sleep Quality

☆ ☆ ☆ ☆ ☆

Weather

- [ ] Sunny ☀
- [ ] Partly Cloudy ☁
- [ ] Cloudy ⛅
- [ ] Windy 🌬
- [ ] Stormy ⛈
- [ ] Light Rain 🌧
- [ ] Heavy Rain 🌧
- [ ] Light Snow 🌨
- [ ] Heavy Snow 🌨
- [ ] Other ....

Mood

- [ ] Happy ☺
- [ ] Calm ☺
- [ ] Confident 😎
- [ ] Excited 😃
- [ ] Loving 😍
- [ ] Other ....
- [ ] Sad ☹
- [ ] Angry 😠
- [ ] Anxious 😟
- [ ] Stressed 😣
- [ ] Self-Critical 😈
- [ ] Tired 😫

Temperature

- [ ] Hot
- [ ] Warm
- [ ] Cold
- [ ] Damp
- [ ] Comfortable

Water

🥛 🥛 🥛 🥛 🥛 🥛 🥛 🥛

Energy Level

☆ ☆ ☆ ☆ ☆

Moon

- [ ] New Moon ●
- [ ] Waxing Crescent ●
- [ ] First Quarter ◐
- [ ] Waxing Gibbous ◑
- [ ] Full Moon ○
- [ ] Waning Gibbous ◑
- [ ] Third Quarter ◑
- [ ] Waning Crescent ◐

Bowel Movement

Constipation   *Diarrhea*

Type 1 Type 2 Type 3 Type 4 Type 5 Type 6 Type 7

Medications

Time	Description

Vitamins

Time	Description

Exercise

Time	Intensity	Activity

Breakfast

Lunch

Dinner

Snacks

Menstrual Cycle Symptoms

- [ ] Cramps
- [ ] Headache
- [ ] Backache
- [ ] Nausea
- [ ] Fatigue
- [ ] Tender Breasts
- [ ] Acne
- [ ] Bloating
- [ ] Cravings
- [ ] Insomnia
- [ ] Other

Physical Symptoms Log

Period

- [ ] Spotting
- [ ] Light
- [ ] Medium
- [ ] Heavy

Pain, Discomfort and Skin Changes

(See the Pain Level Reference and/or Glossary for help in describing your symptoms)

Describe your symptoms, pain level and approximate time in the appropriate space below:

- [ ] Head / Ears / Eyes / Nose / Mouth

- [ ] Throat / Neck

- [ ] Shoulders / Arms / Hands

- [ ] Chest / Heart

- [ ] Back

- [ ] Hips / Buttocks / Legs / Feet

- [ ] Lungs / Breathing (Respiratory)

- [ ] Stomach / Abdomen (Digestive)

- [ ] Uterus / Vagina (Reproductive)

- [ ] Skin

- [ ] Other

Mark all the places on the diagram below that you are experiencing pain, discomfort, and/or skin changes:

Front

Back

Notes

Daily Wellness Log

Date: ....   S M T W Th F Sa

Weight:
Temperature:

Hours of Sleep

0 1 2 3 4 5 6 7 8 9 10 11 12+

Sleep Quality

☆ ☆ ☆ ☆ ☆

Weather

- [ ] Sunny ☀
- [ ] Partly Cloudy ☁
- [ ] Cloudy ⛅
- [ ] Windy 🌬
- [ ] Stormy ⛈
- [ ] Light Rain 🌧
- [ ] Heavy Rain 🌧
- [ ] Light Snow 🌨
- [ ] Heavy Snow 🌨
- [ ] Other ....

Temperature

- [ ] Hot
- [ ] Warm
- [ ] Cold
- [ ] Damp
- [ ] Comfortable

Moon

- [ ] New Moon ●
- [ ] Waxing Crescent ●
- [ ] First Quarter ◐
- [ ] Waxing Gibbous ◑
- [ ] Full Moon ○
- [ ] Waning Gibbous ◑
- [ ] Third Quarter ◑
- [ ] Waning Crescent ●

Mood

- [ ] Happy 😊
- [ ] Calm 🙂
- [ ] Confident 😎
- [ ] Excited 😃
- [ ] Loving 😍
- [ ] Other ....
- [ ] Sad ☹
- [ ] Angry 😠
- [ ] Anxious 😟
- [ ] Stressed 😣
- [ ] Self-Critical 😤
- [ ] Tired 😫

Water

▭ ▭ ▭ ▭ ▭ ▭ ▭ ▭

Energy Level

☆ ☆ ☆ ☆ ☆

Bowel Movement

Constipation   *Diarrhea*

Type 1	Type 2	Type 3	Type 4	Type 5	Type 6	Type 7

Medications

Time	Description

Vitamins

Time	Description

Exercise

Time	Intensity	Activity

Breakfast

Lunch

Dinner

Snacks

Menstrual Cycle Symptoms

☐ Cramps ☐ Headache ☐ Backache ☐ Nausea ☐ Fatigue

☐ Tender Breasts ☐ Acne ☐ Bloating ☐ Cravings ☐ Insomnia

☐ Other _____

Physical Symptoms Log

Period

☐ Spotting ☐ Light ☐ Medium ☐ Heavy

Pain, Discomfort and Skin Changes

(See the Pain Level Reference and/or Glossary for help in describing your symptoms)

Describe your symptoms, pain level and approximate time in the appropriate space below:

☐ Head / Ears / Eyes / Nose / Mouth
_____
_____
_____

☐ Throat / Neck
_____
_____
_____

☐ Shoulders / Arms / Hands
_____
_____
_____

☐ Chest / Heart
_____
_____
_____

☐ Back
_____
_____
_____

☐ Hips / Buttocks / Legs / Feet
_____
_____
_____

☐ Lungs / Breathing (Respiratory)
_____
_____
_____

☐ Stomach / Abdomen (Digestive)
_____
_____
_____

☐ Uterus / Vagina (Reproductive)
_____
_____
_____

☐ Skin
_____
_____
_____

☐ Other
_____
_____
_____

Mark all the places on the diagram below that you are experiencing pain, discomfort, and/or skin changes:

Front

Back

Notes
_____
_____
_____
_____
_____

Daily Wellness Log

Date: ....   S   M   T   W   Th   F   Sa

Weight: _____
Temperature: _____

Hours of Sleep

0   1   2   3   4   5   6   7   8   9   10   11   12+

Sleep Quality

☆ ☆ ☆ ☆ ☆

Weather

- [ ] Sunny ☀
- [ ] Partly Cloudy ☁
- [ ] Cloudy ⛅
- [ ] Windy 🌬
- [ ] Stormy ⛈
- [ ] Light Rain 🌦
- [ ] Heavy Rain 🌧
- [ ] Light Snow 🌨
- [ ] Heavy Snow 🌨
- [ ] Other ....

Mood

- [ ] Happy ☺
- [ ] Calm ☺
- [ ] Confident 😎
- [ ] Excited ☺
- [ ] Loving 😍
- [ ] Other
- [ ] Sad ☹
- [ ] Angry 😠
- [ ] Anxious 😣
- [ ] Stressed 😖
- [ ] Self-Critical 😡
- [ ] Tired 😫

Temperature

- [ ] Hot
- [ ] Warm
- [ ] Cold
- [ ] Damp
- [ ] Comfortable

Water

⬜ ⬜ ⬜ ⬜ ⬜ ⬜ ⬜ ⬜

Energy Level

☆ ☆ ☆ ☆ ☆

Moon

- [ ] New Moon ●
- [ ] Waxing Crescent ●
- [ ] First Quarter ◑
- [ ] Waxing Gibbous ◑
- [ ] Full Moon ○
- [ ] Waning Gibbous ◐
- [ ] Third Quarter ◐
- [ ] Waning Crescent ◐

Bowel Movement

Constipation   *Diarrhea*

Type 1	Type 2	Type 3	Type 4	Type 5	Type 6	Type 7

Medication

Time	Description

Vitamins

Time	Description

Exercise

Time	Intensity	Activity

Breakfast

Lunch

Dinner

Snacks

Menstrual Cycle Symptoms

- [ ] Cramps
- [ ] Headache
- [ ] Backache
- [ ] Nausea
- [ ] Fatigue
- [ ] Tender Breasts
- [ ] Acne
- [ ] Bloating
- [ ] Cravings
- [ ] Insomnia
- [ ] Other

Physical Symptoms Log

Period

- [ ] Spotting
- [ ] Light
- [ ] Medium
- [ ] Heavy

Pain, Discomfort and Skin Changes

(See the Pain Level Reference and/or Glossary for help in describing your symptoms)

Describe your symptoms, pain level and approximate time in the appropriate space below:

- [ ] Head / Ears / Eyes / Nose / Mouth

- [ ] Throat / Neck

- [ ] Shoulders / Arms / Hands

- [ ] Chest / Heart

- [ ] Back

- [ ] Hips / Buttocks / Legs / Feet

- [ ] Lungs / Breathing (Respiratory)

- [ ] Stomach / Abdomen (Digestive)

- [ ] Uterus / Vagina (Reproductive)

- [ ] Skin

- [ ] Other

Mark all the places on the diagram below that you are experiencing pain, discomfort, and/or skin changes:

Front

Back

Notes

Daily Wellness Log

Date: ....

S M T W Th F Sa

Weight:
Temperature:

Hours of Sleep

0 1 2 3 4 5 6 7 8 9 10 11 12+

Sleep Quality

☆ ☆ ☆ ☆ ☆

Weather

- [ ] Sunny ☀
- [ ] Partly Cloudy ☁
- [ ] Cloudy ⛅
- [ ] Windy 🌬
- [ ] Stormy ⛈
- [ ] Light Rain 🌦
- [ ] Heavy Rain 🌧
- [ ] Light Snow 🌨
- [ ] Heavy Snow 🌨
- [ ] Other ....

Mood

- [ ] Happy ☺
- [ ] Calm ☺
- [ ] Confident 😎
- [ ] Excited ☺
- [ ] Loving 😍
- [ ] Other
- [ ] Sad ☹
- [ ] Angry 😠
- [ ] Anxious 😟
- [ ] Stressed 😣
- [ ] Self-Critical 😡
- [ ] Tired 😫

Temperature

- [ ] Hot
- [ ] Warm
- [ ] Cold
- [ ] Damp
- [ ] Comfortable

Water

▽ ▽ ▽ ▽ ▽ ▽ ▽ ▽

Energy Level

☆ ☆ ☆ ☆ ☆

Moon

- [ ] New Moon ●
- [ ] Waxing Crescent ◗
- [ ] First Quarter ◑
- [ ] Waxing Gibbous ◑
- [ ] Full Moon ○
- [ ] Waning Gibbous ◑
- [ ] Third Quarter ◐
- [ ] Waning Crescent ◐

Bowel Movement

Constipation   *Diarrhea*

Type 1	Type 2	Type 3	Type 4	Type 5	Type 6	Type 7

Medications

Time	Description

Vitamins

Time	Description

Exercise

Time	Intensity	Activity

Breakfast

Lunch

Dinner

Snacks

Menstrual Cycle Symptoms

☐ Cramps ☐ Headache ☐ Backache ☐ Nausea ☐ Fatigue

☐ Tender Breasts ☐ Acne ☐ Bloating ☐ Cravings ☐ Insomnia

☐ Other

Physical Symptoms Log

Period

☐ Spotting ☐ Light ☐ Medium ☐ Heavy

Pain, Discomfort and Skin Changes

(See the Pain Level Reference and/or Glossary for help in describing your symptoms)

Describe your symptoms, pain level and approximate time in the appropriate space below:

☐ Head / Ears / Eyes / Nose / Mouth
_____
_____
_____

☐ Throat / Neck
_____
_____

☐ Shoulders / Arms / Hands
_____
_____

☐ Chest / Heart
_____
_____

☐ Back
_____
_____

☐ Hips / Buttocks / Legs / Feet
_____
_____

☐ Lungs / Breathing (Respiratory)
_____
_____

☐ Stomach / Abdomen (Digestive)
_____
_____

☐ Uterus / Vagina (Reproductive)
_____
_____

☐ Skin
_____
_____

☐ Other
_____
_____

Mark all the places on the diagram below that you are experiencing pain, discomfort, and/or skin changes:

Front

Back

Notes

_____
_____
_____
_____

Daily Wellness Log

Date: ....

S M T W Th F Sa

Weight: _____

Temperature: _____

Hours of Sleep

0 1 2 3 4 5 6 7 8 9 10 11 12+

Sleep Quality

☆ ☆ ☆ ☆ ☆

Weather

- [ ] Sunny ☀
- [ ] Partly Cloudy ☁
- [ ] Cloudy ⛅
- [ ] Windy 🌬
- [ ] Stormy ⛈
- [ ] Light Rain 🌦
- [ ] Heavy Rain 🌧
- [ ] Light Snow 🌨
- [ ] Heavy Snow 🌨
- [ ] Other ....

Temperature

- [ ] Hot
- [ ] Warm
- [ ] Cold
- [ ] Damp
- [ ] Comfortable

Mood

- [ ] Happy 😊
- [ ] Calm 🙂
- [ ] Confident 😎
- [ ] Excited 😃
- [ ] Loving 😍
- [ ] Other
- [ ] Sad 😞
- [ ] Angry 😠
- [ ] Anxious 😰
- [ ] Stressed 😣
- [ ] Self-Critical 😤
- [ ] Tired 😫

Water

🥛 🥛 🥛 🥛 🥛 🥛 🥛 🥛

Energy Level

☆ ☆ ☆ ☆ ☆

Moon

- [ ] New Moon ●
- [ ] Waxing Crescent ●
- [ ] First Quarter ◑
- [ ] Waxing Gibbous ◑
- [ ] Full Moon ○
- [ ] Waning Gibbous ◐
- [ ] Third Quarter ◑
- [ ] Waning Crescent ◐

Bowel Movement

Constipation   *Diarrhea*

Type 1   Type 2   Type 3   Type 4   Type 5   Type 6   Type 7

Medications

Time	Description

Vitamins

Time	Description

Exercise

Time	Intensity	Activity

Breakfast

Lunch

Dinner

Snacks

Menstrual Cycle Symptoms

☐ Cramps ☐ Headache ☐ Backache ☐ Nausea ☐ Fatigue

☐ Tender Breasts ☐ Acne ☐ Bloating ☐ Cravings ☐ Insomnia

☐ Other

Physical Symptoms Log

Period

☐ Spotting ☐ Light ☐ Medium ☐ Heavy

Pain, Discomfort and Skin Changes

(See the Pain Level Reference and/or Glossary for help in describing your symptoms)

Describe your symptoms, pain level and approximate time in the appropriate space below:

☐ Head / Ears / Eyes / Nose / Mouth

_____
_____
_____

☐ Shoulders / Arms / Hands

_____
_____
_____

☐ Back

_____
_____
_____

☐ Lungs / Breathing (Respiratory)

_____
_____
_____

☐ Uterus / Vagina (Reproductive)

_____
_____
_____

☐ Other

_____
_____

☐ Throat / Neck

_____
_____
_____

☐ Chest / Heart

_____
_____
_____

☐ Hips / Buttocks / Legs / Feet

_____
_____
_____

☐ Stomach / Abdomen (Digestive)

_____
_____
_____

☐ Skin

_____
_____
_____

Mark all the places on the diagram below that you are experiencing pain, discomfort, and/or skin changes:

Front

Back

Notes

_____
_____
_____
_____

Daily Wellness Log

Date: ....

S M T W Th F Sa

Weight: ....

Temperature: ....

Hours of Sleep

0 1 2 3 4 5 6 7 8 9 10 11 12+

Sleep Quality

☆ ☆ ☆ ☆ ☆

Weather

- [ ] Sunny
- [ ] Partly Cloudy
- [ ] Cloudy
- [ ] Windy
- [ ] Stormy
- [ ] Light Rain
- [ ] Heavy Rain
- [ ] Light Snow
- [ ] Heavy Snow
- [ ] Other ....

Mood

- [ ] Happy
- [ ] Calm
- [ ] Confident
- [ ] Excited
- [ ] Loving
- [ ] Other
- [ ] Sad
- [ ] Angry
- [ ] Anxious
- [ ] Stressed
- [ ] Self-Critical
- [ ] Tired

Temperature

- [ ] Hot
- [ ] Warm
- [ ] Cold
- [ ] Damp
- [ ] Comfortable

Water

Energy Level

☆ ☆ ☆ ☆ ☆

Moon

- [ ] New Moon
- [ ] Waxing Crescent
- [ ] First Quarter
- [ ] Waxing Gibbous
- [ ] Full Moon
- [ ] Waning Gibbous
- [ ] Third Quarter
- [ ] Waning Crescent

Bowel Movement

Constipation   *Diarrhea*

Type 1	Type 2	Type 3	Type 4	Type 5	Type 6	Type 7

Medications

Time	Description

Vitamins

Time	Description

Exercise

Time	Intensity	Activity

Breakfast

Lunch

Dinner

Snacks

Menstrual Cycle Symptoms

- [ ] Cramps
- [ ] Headache
- [ ] Backache
- [ ] Nausea
- [ ] Fatigue
- [ ] Tender Breasts
- [ ] Acne
- [ ] Bloating
- [ ] Cravings
- [ ] Insomnia
- [ ] Other

Physical Symptoms Log

Period

- [ ] Spotting
- [ ] Light
- [ ] Medium
- [ ] Heavy

Pain, Discomfort and Skin Changes

(See the Pain Level Reference and/or Glossary for help in describing your symptoms)

Describe your symptoms, pain level and approximate time in the appropriate space below:

- [ ] Head / Ears / Eyes / Nose / Mouth

- [ ] Throat / Neck

- [ ] Shoulders / Arms / Hands

- [ ] Chest / Heart

- [ ] Back

- [ ] Hips / Buttocks / Legs / Feet

- [ ] Lungs / Breathing (Respiratory)

- [ ] Stomach / Abdomen (Digestive)

- [ ] Uterus / Vagina (Reproductive)

- [ ] Skin

- [ ] Other

Mark all the places on the diagram below that you are experiencing pain, discomfort, and/or skin changes:

Front

Back

Notes

Daily Wellness Log

Date: ....   S   M   T   W   Th   F   Sa

Weight:

Temperature:

Hours of Sleep

0   1   2   3   4   5   6   7   8   9   10   11   12+

Sleep Quality

☆ ☆ ☆ ☆ ☆

Weather

- [ ] Sunny ☀
- [ ] Partly Cloudy ☁
- [ ] Cloudy ⛅
- [ ] Windy 🌬
- [ ] Stormy ⚡
- [ ] Light Rain 🌧
- [ ] Heavy Rain 🌧
- [ ] Light Snow 🌨
- [ ] Heavy Snow 🌨
- [ ] Other ....

Mood

- [ ] Happy ☺
- [ ] Calm ☺
- [ ] Confident 😎
- [ ] Excited ☺
- [ ] Loving 😍
- [ ] Other ....
- [ ] Sad ☹
- [ ] Angry 😠
- [ ] Anxious 😰
- [ ] Stressed 😖
- [ ] Self-Critical 😈
- [ ] Tired 😫

Temperature

- [ ] Hot
- [ ] Warm
- [ ] Cold
- [ ] Damp
- [ ] Comfortable

Water

🥛 🥛 🥛 🥛 🥛 🥛 🥛 🥛

Energy Level

☆ ☆ ☆ ☆ ☆

Moon

- [ ] New Moon ●
- [ ] Waxing Crescent ●
- [ ] First Quarter ◑
- [ ] Waxing Gibbous ◑
- [ ] Full Moon ○
- [ ] Waning Gibbous ◑
- [ ] Third Quarter ◑
- [ ] Waning Crescent ●

Bowel Movement

Constipation   *Diarrhea*

Type 1	Type 2	Type 3	Type 4	Type 5	Type 6	Type 7

Medications

Time	Description

Vitamins

Time	Description

Exercise

Time	Intensity	Activity

Breakfast

Lunch

Dinner

Snacks

Menstrual Cycle Symptoms

- [ ] Cramps
- [ ] Headache
- [ ] Backache
- [ ] Nausea
- [ ] Fatigue
- [ ] Tender Breasts
- [ ] Acne
- [ ] Bloating
- [ ] Cravings
- [ ] Insomnia
- [ ] Other

Physical Symptoms Log

Period

- [ ] Spotting
- [ ] Light
- [ ] Medium
- [ ] Heavy

Pain, Discomfort and Skin Changes

(See the Pain Level Reference and/or Glossary for help in describing your symptoms)

Describe your symptoms, pain level and approximate time in the appropriate space below:

- [ ] Head / Ears / Eyes / Nose / Mouth
- [ ] Throat / Neck
- [ ] Shoulders / Arms / Hands
- [ ] Chest / Heart
- [ ] Back
- [ ] Hips / Buttocks / Legs / Feet
- [ ] Lungs / Breathing (Respiratory)
- [ ] Stomach / Abdomen (Digestive)
- [ ] Uterus / Vagina (Reproductive)
- [ ] Skin
- [ ] Other

Mark all the places on the diagram below that you are experiencing pain, discomfort, and/or skin changes:

Front

Back

Notes

Daily Wellness Log

Date: ....

S M T W Th F Sa

Weight: _____
Temperature: _____

Hours of Sleep

0 1 2 3 4 5 6 7 8 9 10 11 12+

Sleep Quality

☆ ☆ ☆ ☆ ☆

Weather

- ☐ Sunny ☀
- ☐ Partly Cloudy ☁
- ☐ Cloudy ⛅
- ☐ Windy 🌬
- ☐ Stormy ⛈
- ☐ Light Rain 🌦
- ☐ Heavy Rain 🌧
- ☐ Light Snow 🌨
- ☐ Heavy Snow 🌨
- ☐ Other ....

Mood

- ☐ Happy ☺
- ☐ Calm ☺
- ☐ Confident 😎
- ☐ Excited ☺
- ☐ Loving 😍
- ☐ Other
- ☐ Sad ☹
- ☐ Angry 😠
- ☐ Anxious 😧
- ☐ Stressed 😖
- ☐ Self-Critical 😡
- ☐ Tired 😫

Temperature

☐ Hot ☐ Warm ☐ Cold ☐ Damp ☐ Comfortable

Water

🥛 🥛 🥛 🥛 🥛 🥛 🥛 🥛

Energy Level

☆ ☆ ☆ ☆ ☆

Moon

- ☐ New Moon ●
- ☐ Waxing Crescent ◐
- ☐ First Quarter ◑
- ☐ Waxing Gibbous ◑
- ☐ Full Moon ○
- ☐ Waning Gibbous ◑
- ☐ Third Quarter ◐
- ☐ Waning Crescent ◐

Bowel Movement

Constipation   *Diarrhea*

Type 1	Type 2	Type 3	Type 4	Type 5	Type 6	Type 7

Medications

Time	Description

Vitamins

Time	Description

Exercise

Time	Intensity	Activity

Breakfast

Lunch

Dinner

Snacks

Menstrual Cycle Symptoms

☐ Cramps ☐ Headache ☐ Backache ☐ Nausea ☐ Fatigue

☐ Tender Breasts ☐ Acne ☐ Bloating ☐ Cravings ☐ Insomnia

☐ Other

Physical Symptoms Log

Period

☐ Spotting ☐ Light ☐ Medium ☐ Heavy

Pain, Discomfort and Skin Changes

(See the Pain Level Reference and/or Glossary for help in describing your symptoms)

Describe your symptoms, pain level and approximate time in the appropriate space below:

☐ Head / Ears / Eyes / Nose / Mouth

_____
_____
_____

☐ Shoulders / Arms / Hands

_____
_____

☐ Back

_____
_____
_____

☐ Lungs / Breathing (Respiratory)

_____
_____

☐ Uterus / Vagina (Reproductive)

_____
_____
_____

☐ Other

_____
_____

☐ Throat / Neck

_____
_____
_____

☐ Chest / Heart

_____
_____

☐ Hips / Buttocks / Legs / Feet

_____
_____
_____

☐ Stomach / Abdomen (Digestive)

_____
_____

☐ Skin

_____
_____

Mark all the places on the diagram below that you are experiencing pain, discomfort, and/or skin changes:

Front

Back

Notes

_____
_____
_____
_____

Daily Wellness Log

Date: ....

S M T W Th F Sa

Weight: ....
Temperature: ....

Hours of Sleep

0 1 2 3 4 5 6 7 8 9 10 11 12+

Sleep Quality

☆ ☆ ☆ ☆ ☆

Weather

- [ ] Sunny ☀
- [ ] Partly Cloudy ☁
- [ ] Cloudy ⛅
- [ ] Windy 🌬
- [ ] Stormy ⛈
- [ ] Light Rain 🌦
- [ ] Heavy Rain 🌧
- [ ] Light Snow 🌨
- [ ] Heavy Snow 🌨
- [ ] Other ....

Mood

- [ ] Happy ☺
- [ ] Calm ☺
- [ ] Confident 😎
- [ ] Excited 😃
- [ ] Loving 😍
- [ ] Other
- [ ] Sad ☹
- [ ] Angry 😠
- [ ] Anxious 😟
- [ ] Stressed 😖
- [ ] Self-Critical 😣
- [ ] Tired 😫

Temperature

- [ ] Hot
- [ ] Warm
- [ ] Cold
- [ ] Damp
- [ ] Comfortable

Water

🥛 🥛 🥛 🥛 🥛 🥛 🥛 🥛

Energy Level

☆ ☆ ☆ ☆ ☆

Moon

- [ ] New Moon ●
- [ ] Waxing Crescent ●
- [ ] First Quarter ◑
- [ ] Waxing Gibbous ◑
- [ ] Full Moon ○
- [ ] Waning Gibbous ◐
- [ ] Third Quarter ◐
- [ ] Waning Crescent ◐

Bowel Movement

Constipation   *Diarrhea*

Type 1	Type 2	Type 3	Type 4	Type 5	Type 6	Type 7

Medications

Time	Description

Vitamins

Time	Description

Exercise

Time	Intensity	Activity

Breakfast

Lunch

Dinner

Snacks

Menstrual Cycle Symptoms

- [ ] Cramps
- [ ] Headache
- [ ] Backache
- [ ] Nausea
- [ ] Fatigue
- [ ] Tender Breasts
- [ ] Acne
- [ ] Bloating
- [ ] Cravings
- [ ] Insomnia
- [ ] Other

Physical Symptoms Log

Period

- [ ] Spotting
- [ ] Light
- [ ] Medium
- [ ] Heavy

Pain, Discomfort and Skin Changes

(See the Pain Level Reference and/or Glossary for help in describing your symptoms)

Describe your symptoms, pain level and approximate time in the appropriate space below:

- [ ] Head / Ears / Eyes / Nose / Mouth

- [ ] Throat / Neck

- [ ] Shoulders / Arms / Hands

- [ ] Chest / Heart

- [ ] Back

- [ ] Hips / Buttocks / Legs / Feet

- [ ] Lungs / Breathing (Respiratory)

- [ ] Stomach / Abdomen (Digestive)

- [ ] Uterus / Vagina (Reproductive)

- [ ] Skin

- [ ] Other

Mark all the places on the diagram below that you are experiencing pain, discomfort, and/or skin changes:

Front

Back

Notes

Daily Wellness Log

Date: ....

S M T W Th F Sa

Weight: ....

Temperature: ....

Hours of Sleep

0 1 2 3 4 5 6 7 8 9 10 11 12+

Sleep Quality

☆ ☆ ☆ ☆ ☆

Weather

- [ ] Sunny
- [ ] Partly Cloudy
- [ ] Cloudy
- [ ] Windy
- [ ] Stormy
- [ ] Light Rain
- [ ] Heavy Rain
- [ ] Light Snow
- [ ] Heavy Snow
- [ ] Other ....

Mood

- [ ] Happy
- [ ] Calm
- [ ] Confident
- [ ] Excited
- [ ] Loving
- [ ] Other
- [ ] Sad
- [ ] Angry
- [ ] Anxious
- [ ] Stressed
- [ ] Self-Critical
- [ ] Tired

Temperature

- [ ] Hot
- [ ] Warm
- [ ] Cold
- [ ] Damp
- [ ] Comfortable

Water

🥛 🥛 🥛 🥛 🥛 🥛 🥛 🥛

Energy Level

☆ ☆ ☆ ☆ ☆

Moon

- [ ] New Moon
- [ ] Waxing Crescent
- [ ] First Quarter
- [ ] Waxing Gibbous
- [ ] Full Moon
- [ ] Waning Gibbous
- [ ] Third Quarter
- [ ] Waning Crescent

Bowel Movement

Constipation | | | | | | Diarrhea

Type 1 | Type 2 | Type 3 | Type 4 | Type 5 | Type 6 | Type 7

Medications

Time	Description

Vitamins

Time	Description

Exercise

Time	Intensity	Activity

Breakfast

Lunch

Dinner

Snacks

Menstrual Cycle Symptoms

☐ Cramps   ☐ Headache   ☐ Backache   ☐ Nausea   ☐ Fatigue

☐ Tender Breasts   ☐ Acne   ☐ Bloating   ☐ Cravings   ☐ Insomnia

☐ Other ....

Physical Symptoms Log

Period

☐ Spotting   ☐ Light   ☐ Medium   ☐ Heavy

Pain, Discomfort and Skin Changes

(See the Pain Level Reference and/or Glossary for help in describing your symptoms)

Describe your symptoms, pain level and approximate time in the appropriate space below:

☐ Head / Ears / Eyes / Nose / Mouth
_____
_____
_____

☐ Throat / Neck
_____
_____
_____

☐ Shoulders / Arms / Hands
_____
_____
_____

☐ Chest / Heart
_____
_____
_____

☐ Back
_____
_____
_____

☐ Hips / Buttocks / Legs / Feet
_____
_____
_____

☐ Lungs / Breathing (Respiratory)
_____
_____

☐ Stomach / Abdomen (Digestive)
_____
_____

☐ Uterus / Vagina (Reproductive)
_____
_____
_____

☐ Skin
_____
_____
_____

☐ Other
_____
_____

Mark all the places on the diagram below that you are experiencing pain, discomfort, and/or skin changes:

Front

Back

Notes
_____
_____
_____
_____

Daily Wellness Log

Date: ....   S M T W Th F Sa

Weight: _____
Temperature: _____

Hours of Sleep

0 1 2 3 4 5 6 7 8 9 10 11 12+

Sleep Quality
☆ ☆ ☆ ☆ ☆

Weather
- [ ] Sunny ☀
- [ ] Partly Cloudy ☁
- [ ] Cloudy ⛅
- [ ] Windy 🌫
- [ ] Stormy ⛈
- [ ] Light Rain 🌧
- [ ] Heavy Rain 🌧
- [ ] Light Snow 🌨
- [ ] Heavy Snow 🌨
- [ ] Other ....

Mood
- [ ] Happy ☺
- [ ] Calm ☺
- [ ] Confident 😎
- [ ] Excited 😀
- [ ] Loving 😍
- [ ] Other
- [ ] Sad ☹
- [ ] Angry ☹
- [ ] Anxious ☹
- [ ] Stressed 😖
- [ ] Self-Critical 😠
- [ ] Tired 😫

Temperature
- [ ] Hot
- [ ] Warm
- [ ] Cold
- [ ] Damp
- [ ] Comfortable

Water
⛾ ⛾ ⛾ ⛾ ⛾ ⛾ ⛾ ⛾

Energy Level
☆ ☆ ☆ ☆ ☆

Moon
- [ ] New Moon ⬤
- [ ] Waxing Crescent ⬤
- [ ] First Quarter ◑
- [ ] Waxing Gibbous ◑
- [ ] Full Moon ○
- [ ] Waning Gibbous ◐
- [ ] Third Quarter ◐
- [ ] Waning Crescent ◑

Bowel Movement

Constipation   *Diarrhea*

Type 1	Type 2	Type 3	Type 4	Type 5	Type 6	Type 7

Medications

Time	Description

Vitamins

Time	Description

Exercise

Time	Intensity	Activity

Breakfast

Lunch

Dinner

Snacks

Menstrual Cycle Symptoms

☐ Cramps ☐ Headache ☐ Backache ☐ Nausea ☐ Fatigue

☐ Tender Breasts ☐ Acne ☐ Bloating ☐ Cravings ☐ Insomnia

☐ Other

Physical Symptoms Log

Period

☐ Spotting ☐ Light ☐ Medium ☐ Heavy

Pain, Discomfort and Skin Changes

(See the Pain Level Reference and/or Glossary for help in describing your symptoms)

Describe your symptoms, pain level and approximate time in the appropriate space below:

☐ Head / Ears / Eyes / Nose / Mouth

_____
_____
_____

☐ Throat / Neck

_____
_____
_____

☐ Shoulders / Arms / Hands

_____
_____
_____

☐ Chest / Heart

_____
_____
_____

☐ Back

_____
_____
_____

☐ Hips / Buttocks / Legs / Feet

_____
_____
_____

☐ Lungs / Breathing (Respiratory)

_____
_____
_____

☐ Stomach / Abdomen (Digestive)

_____
_____
_____

☐ Uterus / Vagina (Reproductive)

_____
_____
_____

☐ Skin

_____
_____
_____

☐ Other

_____
_____
_____

Mark all the places on the diagram below that you are experiencing pain, discomfort, and/or skin changes:

Front

Back

Notes

_____
_____
_____
_____

Daily Wellness Log

Date: ....

S M T W Th F Sa

Weight: _____
Temperature: _____

Hours of Sleep

0 1 2 3 4 5 6 7 8 9 10 11 12+

Sleep Quality

☆ ☆ ☆ ☆ ☆

Weather

- [ ] Sunny ☀
- [ ] Partly Cloudy ☁
- [ ] Cloudy ⛅
- [ ] Windy 🌬
- [ ] Stormy ⛈
- [ ] Light Rain 🌦
- [ ] Heavy Rain 🌧
- [ ] Light Snow 🌨
- [ ] Heavy Snow 🌨
- [ ] Other ....

Mood

- [ ] Happy 🙂
- [ ] Calm 🙂
- [ ] Confident 😎
- [ ] Excited 😃
- [ ] Loving 😍
- [ ] Other
- [ ] Sad ☹
- [ ] Angry 😠
- [ ] Anxious 😟
- [ ] Stressed 😣
- [ ] Self-Critical 😖
- [ ] Tired 😫

Temperature

- [ ] Hot
- [ ] Warm
- [ ] Cold
- [ ] Damp
- [ ] Comfortable

Water

🥛 🥛 🥛 🥛 🥛 🥛 🥛 🥛

Energy Level

☆ ☆ ☆ ☆ ☆

Moon

- [ ] New Moon ●
- [ ] Waxing Crescent ◐
- [ ] First Quarter ◑
- [ ] Waxing Gibbous ◑
- [ ] Full Moon ○
- [ ] Waning Gibbous ◐
- [ ] Third Quarter ◑
- [ ] Waning Crescent ◐

Bowel Movement

Constipation   *Diarrhea*

Type 1	Type 2	Type 3	Type 4	Type 5	Type 6	Type 7

Medications

Time	Description

Vitamins

Time	Description

Exercise

Time	Intensity	Activity

Breakfast

Lunch

Dinner

Snacks

Menstrual Cycle Symptoms

- [ ] Cramps
- [ ] Headache
- [ ] Backache
- [ ] Nausea
- [ ] Fatigue
- [ ] Tender Breasts
- [ ] Acne
- [ ] Bloating
- [ ] Cravings
- [ ] Insomnia
- [ ] Other

Physical Symptoms Log

Period

- [ ] Spotting
- [ ] Light
- [ ] Medium
- [ ] Heavy

Pain, Discomfort and Skin Changes

(See the Pain Level Reference and/or Glossary for help in describing your symptoms)

Describe your symptoms, pain level and approximate time in the appropriate space below:

- [ ] Head / Ears / Eyes / Nose / Mouth

- [ ] Throat / Neck

- [ ] Shoulders / Arms / Hands

- [ ] Chest / Heart

- [ ] Back

- [ ] Hips / Buttocks / Legs / Feet

- [ ] Lungs / Breathing (Respiratory)

- [ ] Stomach / Abdomen (Digestive)

- [ ] Uterus / Vagina (Reproductive)

- [ ] Skin

- [ ] Other

Mark all the places on the diagram below that you are experiencing pain, discomfort, and/or skin changes:

Front

Back

Notes

Daily Wellness Log

Date: ....   S M T W Th F Sa

Weight: ....
Temperature: ....

Hours of Sleep

0   1   2   3   4   5   6   7   8   9   10   11   12+

Sleep Quality

☆ ☆ ☆ ☆ ☆

Weather

- [ ] Sunny ☀
- [ ] Partly Cloudy ☁
- [ ] Cloudy ⛅
- [ ] Windy 🌬
- [ ] Stormy ⛈
- [ ] Light Rain 🌦
- [ ] Heavy Rain 🌧
- [ ] Light Snow 🌨
- [ ] Heavy Snow 🌨
- [ ] Other ....

Mood

- [ ] Happy 🙂
- [ ] Calm 🙂
- [ ] Confident 😎
- [ ] Excited 😀
- [ ] Loving 😍
- [ ] Other
- [ ] Sad ☹
- [ ] Angry 😠
- [ ] Anxious 😣
- [ ] Stressed 😖
- [ ] Self-Critical 😤
- [ ] Tired 😫

Temperature

- [ ] Hot
- [ ] Warm
- [ ] Cold
- [ ] Damp
- [ ] Comfortable

Water

⊔ ⊔ ⊔ ⊔ ⊔ ⊔ ⊔ ⊔

Energy Level

☆ ☆ ☆ ☆ ☆

Moon

- [ ] New Moon ●
- [ ] Waxing Crescent ●
- [ ] First Quarter ◑
- [ ] Waxing Gibbous ◑
- [ ] Full Moon ○
- [ ] Waning Gibbous ◐
- [ ] Third Quarter ◐
- [ ] Waning Crescent ●

Bowel Movement

Constipation   *Diarrhea*

Type 1	Type 2	Type 3	Type 4	Type 5	Type 6	Type 7

Medications

Time	Description

Vitamins

Time	Description

Exercise

Time	Intensity	Activity

Breakfast

Lunch

Dinner

Snacks

Menstrual Cycle Symptoms

- ☐ Cramps
- ☐ Headache
- ☐ Backache
- ☐ Nausea
- ☐ Fatigue
- ☐ Tender Breasts
- ☐ Acne
- ☐ Bloating
- ☐ Cravings
- ☐ Insomnia
- ☐ Other

Physical Symptoms Log

Period

- ☐ Spotting
- ☐ Light
- ☐ Medium
- ☐ Heavy

Pain, Discomfort and Skin Changes

(See the Pain Level Reference and/or Glossary for help in describing your symptoms)

Describe your symptoms, pain level and approximate time in the appropriate space below:

☐ Head / Ears / Eyes / Nose / Mouth

☐ Throat / Neck

☐ Shoulders / Arms / Hands

☐ Chest / Heart

☐ Back

☐ Hips / Buttocks / Legs / Feet

☐ Lungs / Breathing (Respiratory)

☐ Stomach / Abdomen (Digestive)

☐ Uterus / Vagina (Reproductive)

☐ Skin

☐ Other

Mark all the places on the diagram below that you are experiencing pain, discomfort, and/or skin changes:

Front

Back

Notes

Daily Wellness Log

Date: ....   S M T W Th F Sa

Weight: _____
Temperature: _____

Hours of Sleep

0   1   2   3   4   5   6   7   8   9   10   11   12+

Sleep Quality
☆ ☆ ☆ ☆ ☆

Weather
- ☐ Sunny ☀
- ☐ Partly Cloudy ☁
- ☐ Cloudy ⛅
- ☐ Windy 🌬
- ☐ Stormy ⛈
- ☐ Light Rain 🌦
- ☐ Heavy Rain 🌧
- ☐ Light Snow 🌨
- ☐ Heavy Snow 🌨
- ☐ Other ....

Mood
- ☐ Happy 🙂
- ☐ Calm 🙂
- ☐ Confident 😎
- ☐ Excited 😃
- ☐ Loving 😍
- ☐ Other
- ☐ Sad ☹
- ☐ Angry 😠
- ☐ Anxious 😧
- ☐ Stressed 😣
- ☐ Self-Critical 😖
- ☐ Tired 😫

Temperature
- ☐ Hot
- ☐ Warm
- ☐ Cold
- ☐ Damp
- ☐ Comfortable

Water
▽ ▽ ▽ ▽ ▽ ▽ ▽ ▽

Energy Level
☆ ☆ ☆ ☆ ☆

Moon
- ☐ New Moon ●
- ☐ Waxing Crescent ●
- ☐ First Quarter ◑
- ☐ Waxing Gibbous ◑
- ☐ Full Moon ○
- ☐ Waning Gibbous ◐
- ☐ Third Quarter ◐
- ☐ Waning Crescent ◐

Bowel Movement

Constipation   Diarrhea

Type 1	Type 2	Type 3	Type 4	Type 5	Type 6	Type 7

Medications

Time	Description

Vitamins

Time	Description

Exercise

Time	Intensity	Activity

Breakfast

Lunch

Dinner

Snacks

Menstrual Cycle Symptoms

- [ ] Cramps
- [ ] Headache
- [ ] Backache
- [ ] Nausea
- [ ] Fatigue
- [ ] Tender Breasts
- [ ] Acne
- [ ] Bloating
- [ ] Cravings
- [ ] Insomnia
- [ ] Other

Physical Symptoms Log

Period

- [ ] Spotting
- [ ] Light
- [ ] Medium
- [ ] Heavy

Pain, Discomfort and Skin Changes

(See the Pain Level Reference and/or Glossary for help in describing your symptoms)

Describe your symptoms, pain level and approximate time in the appropriate space below:

- [ ] Head / Ears / Eyes / Nose / Mouth

- [ ] Throat / Neck

- [ ] Shoulders / Arms / Hands

- [ ] Chest / Heart

- [ ] Back

- [ ] Hips / Buttocks / Legs / Feet

- [ ] Lungs / Breathing (Respiratory)

- [ ] Stomach / Abdomen (Digestive)

- [ ] Uterus / Vagina (Reproductive)

- [ ] Skin

- [ ] Other

Mark all the places on the diagram below that you are experiencing pain, discomfort, and/or skin changes:

Front

Back

Notes

Daily Wellness Log

Date: ....

S M T W Th F Sa

Weight:
Temperature:

Hours of Sleep

0 1 2 3 4 5 6 7 8 9 10 11 12+

Sleep Quality

☆ ☆ ☆ ☆ ☆

Weather

- ☐ Sunny ☀
- ☐ Partly Cloudy ☁
- ☐ Cloudy ⛅
- ☐ Windy 🌬
- ☐ Stormy ⛈
- ☐ Light Rain 🌧
- ☐ Heavy Rain 🌧
- ☐ Light Snow 🌨
- ☐ Heavy Snow 🌨
- ☐ Other ....

Mood

- ☐ Happy ☺
- ☐ Calm ☺
- ☐ Confident 😎
- ☐ Excited 😃
- ☐ Loving 😍
- ☐ Other
- ☐ Sad ☹
- ☐ Angry 😠
- ☐ Anxious 😟
- ☐ Stressed 😖
- ☐ Self-Critical 😣
- ☐ Tired 😫

Temperature

☐ Hot   ☐ Warm   ☐ Cold   ☐ Damp   ☐ Comfortable

Water

🥤 🥤 🥤 🥤 🥤 🥤 🥤 🥤

Energy Level

☆ ☆ ☆ ☆ ☆

Moon

- ☐ New Moon ●
- ☐ Waxing Crescent ●
- ☐ First Quarter ◑
- ☐ Waxing Gibbous ◗
- ☐ Full Moon ○
- ☐ Waning Gibbous ◖
- ☐ Third Quarter ◐
- ☐ Waning Crescent ◕

Bowel Movement

Constipation   *Diarrhea*

Type 1	Type 2	Type 3	Type 4	Type 5	Type 6	Type 7

Medications

Time	Description

Vitamins

Time	Description

Exercise

Time	Intensity	Activity

Breakfast

Lunch

Dinner

Snacks

Menstrual Cycle Symptoms

- ☐ Cramps
- ☐ Headache
- ☐ Backache
- ☐ Nausea
- ☐ Fatigue
- ☐ Tender Breasts
- ☐ Acne
- ☐ Bloating
- ☐ Cravings
- ☐ Insomnia
- ☐ Other

Physical Symptoms Log

Period

- ☐ Spotting
- ☐ Light
- ☐ Medium
- ☐ Heavy

Pain, Discomfort and Skin Changes

(See the Pain Level Reference and/or Glossary for help in describing your symptoms)

Describe your symptoms, pain level and approximate time in the appropriate space below:

☐ Head / Ears / Eyes / Nose / Mouth

☐ Throat / Neck

☐ Shoulders / Arms / Hands

☐ Chest / Heart

☐ Back

☐ Hips / Buttocks / Legs / Feet

☐ Lungs / Breathing (Respiratory)

☐ Stomach / Abdomen (Digestive)

☐ Uterus / Vagina (Reproductive)

☐ Skin

☐ Other

Mark all the places on the diagram below that you are experiencing pain, discomfort, and/or skin changes:

Front

Back

Notes

Daily Wellness Log

Date: ....

S M T W Th F Sa

Weight:
Temperature:

Hours of Sleep

0 1 2 3 4 5 6 7 8 9 10 11 12+

Sleep Quality

☆ ☆ ☆ ☆ ☆

Weather

- [ ] Sunny ☀
- [ ] Partly Cloudy ☁
- [ ] Cloudy ⛅
- [ ] Windy 🌬
- [ ] Stormy ⛈
- [ ] Light Rain 🌧
- [ ] Heavy Rain 🌧
- [ ] Light Snow 🌨
- [ ] Heavy Snow 🌨
- [ ] Other ....

Mood

- [ ] Happy 🙂
- [ ] Calm 🙂
- [ ] Confident 😎
- [ ] Excited 😄
- [ ] Loving 😍
- [ ] Other ....
- [ ] Sad ☹
- [ ] Angry 😠
- [ ] Anxious 😧
- [ ] Stressed 😖
- [ ] Self-Critical 😤
- [ ] Tired 😫

Temperature

- [ ] Hot
- [ ] Warm
- [ ] Cold
- [ ] Damp
- [ ] Comfortable

Water

🥛 🥛 🥛 🥛 🥛 🥛 🥛 🥛

Energy Level

☆ ☆ ☆ ☆ ☆

Moon

- [ ] New Moon ●
- [ ] Waxing Crescent ●
- [ ] First Quarter ◐
- [ ] Waxing Gibbous ◑
- [ ] Full Moon ○
- [ ] Waning Gibbous ◑
- [ ] Third Quarter ◐
- [ ] Waning Crescent ◑

Bowel Movement

Constipation   *Diarrhea*

Type 1	Type 2	Type 3	Type 4	Type 5	Type 6	Type 7

Medications

Time	Description

Vitamins

Time	Description

Exercise

Time	Intensity	Activity

Breakfast

Lunch

Dinner

Snacks

Menstrual Cycle Symptoms

☐ Cramps ☐ Headache ☐ Backache ☐ Nausea ☐ Fatigue

☐ Tender Breasts ☐ Acne ☐ Bloating ☐ Cravings ☐ Insomnia

☐ Other

Physical Symptoms Log

Period

☐ Spotting ☐ Light ☐ Medium ☐ Heavy

Pain, Discomfort and Skin Changes

(See the Pain Level Reference and/or Glossary for help in describing your symptoms)

Describe your symptoms, pain level and approximate time in the appropriate space below:

☐ Head / Ears / Eyes / Nose / Mouth

☐ Throat / Neck

☐ Shoulders / Arms / Hands

☐ Chest / Heart

☐ Back

☐ Hips / Buttocks / Legs / Feet

☐ Lungs / Breathing (Respiratory)

☐ Stomach / Abdomen (Digestive)

☐ Uterus / Vagina (Reproductive)

☐ Skin

☐ Other

Mark all the places on the diagram below that you are experiencing pain, discomfort, and/or skin changes:

Front

Back

Notes

Daily Wellness Log

Date: ....   S M T W Th F Sa

Weight:
Temperature:

Hours of Sleep

0 1 2 3 4 5 6 7 8 9 10 11 12+

Sleep Quality

☆ ☆ ☆ ☆ ☆

Weather

- [ ] Sunny ☀
- [ ] Partly Cloudy ☁
- [ ] Cloudy ⛅
- [ ] Windy 🌬
- [ ] Stormy ⛈
- [ ] Light Rain 🌧
- [ ] Heavy Rain 🌧
- [ ] Light Snow 🌨
- [ ] Heavy Snow 🌨
- [ ] Other ....

Mood

- [ ] Happy 🙂
- [ ] Calm 🙂
- [ ] Confident 😎
- [ ] Excited 😀
- [ ] Loving 😍
- [ ] Other
- [ ] Sad ☹
- [ ] Angry 😠
- [ ] Anxious 😖
- [ ] Stressed 😣
- [ ] Self-Critical 😤
- [ ] Tired 😫

Temperature

- [ ] Hot
- [ ] Warm
- [ ] Cold
- [ ] Damp
- [ ] Comfortable

Water

⊔ ⊔ ⊔ ⊔ ⊔ ⊔ ⊔ ⊔

Energy Level

☆ ☆ ☆ ☆ ☆

Moon

- [ ] New Moon ●
- [ ] Waxing Crescent ●
- [ ] First Quarter ◐
- [ ] Waxing Gibbous ◔
- [ ] Full Moon ○
- [ ] Waning Gibbous ◑
- [ ] Third Quarter ◑
- [ ] Waning Crescent ◕

Bowel Movement

Constipation   *Diarrhea*

Type 1	Type 2	Type 3	Type 4	Type 5	Type 6	Type 7

Medications

Time	Description

Vitamins

Time	Description

Exercise

Time	Intensity	Activity

Breakfast

Lunch

Dinner

Snacks

Menstrual Cycle Symptoms

- [ ] Cramps
- [ ] Headache
- [ ] Backache
- [ ] Nausea
- [ ] Fatigue
- [ ] Tender Breasts
- [ ] Acne
- [ ] Bloating
- [ ] Cravings
- [ ] Insomnia
- [ ] Other

Physical Symptoms Log

Period

- [ ] Spotting
- [ ] Light
- [ ] Medium
- [ ] Heavy

Pain, Discomfort and Skin Changes

(See the Pain Level Reference and/or Glossary for help in describing your symptoms)

Describe your symptoms, pain level and approximate time in the appropriate space below:

- [ ] Head / Ears / Eyes / Nose / Mouth
- [ ] Throat / Neck
- [ ] Shoulders / Arms / Hands
- [ ] Chest / Heart
- [ ] Back
- [ ] Hips / Buttocks / Legs / Feet
- [ ] Lungs / Breathing (Respiratory)
- [ ] Stomach / Abdomen (Digestive)
- [ ] Uterus / Vagina (Reproductive)
- [ ] Skin
- [ ] Other

Mark all the places on the diagram below that you are experiencing pain, discomfort, and/or skin changes:

Front

Back

Notes

Daily Wellness Log

Date: ....   S   M   T   W   Th   F   Sa

Weight: ....
Temperature: ....

Hours of Sleep

0   1   2   3   4   5   6   7   8   9   10   11   12+

Sleep Quality

☆ ☆ ☆ ☆ ☆

Weather

- [ ] Sunny ☀
- [ ] Partly Cloudy ☁
- [ ] Cloudy ⛅
- [ ] Windy 🌫
- [ ] Stormy ⛈
- [ ] Light Rain 🌧
- [ ] Heavy Rain 🌧
- [ ] Light Snow 🌨
- [ ] Heavy Snow 🌨
- [ ] Other ....

Mood

- [ ] Happy 😊
- [ ] Calm 🙂
- [ ] Confident 😎
- [ ] Excited 😄
- [ ] Loving 😍
- [ ] Other ....
- [ ] Sad ☹
- [ ] Angry 😠
- [ ] Anxious 😧
- [ ] Stressed 😫
- [ ] Self-Critical 😣
- [ ] Tired 😫

Temperature

- [ ] Hot [ ] Warm [ ] Cold [ ] Damp [ ] Comfortable

Water

⊔ ⊔ ⊔ ⊔ ⊔ ⊔ ⊔ ⊔

Energy Level

☆ ☆ ☆ ☆ ☆

Moon

- [ ] New Moon ●
- [ ] Waxing Crescent ◐
- [ ] First Quarter ◐
- [ ] Waxing Gibbous ◑
- [ ] Full Moon ○
- [ ] Waning Gibbous ◑
- [ ] Third Quarter ◐
- [ ] Waning Crescent ◑

Bowel Movement

Constipation   *Diarrhea*

Type 1	Type 2	Type 3	Type 4	Type 5	Type 6	Type 7

Medications

Time	Description

Vitamins

Time	Description

Exercise

Time	Intensity	Activity

Breakfast

Lunch

Dinner

Snacks

Menstrual Cycle Symptoms

- [ ] Cramps
- [ ] Headache
- [ ] Backache
- [ ] Nausea
- [ ] Fatigue
- [ ] Tender Breasts
- [ ] Acne
- [ ] Bloating
- [ ] Cravings
- [ ] Insomnia
- [ ] Other

Physical Symptoms Log

Period

- [ ] Spotting
- [ ] Light
- [ ] Medium
- [ ] Heavy

Pain, Discomfort and Skin Changes

(See the Pain Level Reference and/or Glossary for help in describing your symptoms)

Describe your symptoms, pain level and approximate time in the appropriate space below:

- [ ] Head / Ears / Eyes / Nose / Mouth

- [ ] Throat / Neck

- [ ] Shoulders / Arms / Hands

- [ ] Chest / Heart

- [ ] Back

- [ ] Hips / Buttocks / Legs / Feet

- [ ] Lungs / Breathing (Respiratory)

- [ ] Stomach / Abdomen (Digestive)

- [ ] Uterus / Vagina (Reproductive)

- [ ] Skin

- [ ] Other

Mark all the places on the diagram below that you are experiencing pain, discomfort, and/or skin changes:

Front

Back

Notes

Daily Wellness Log

Date: ....   S M T W Th F Sa

Weight:
Temperature:

Hours of Sleep

0 1 2 3 4 5 6 7 8 9 10 11 12+

Sleep Quality

☆ ☆ ☆ ☆ ☆

Weather

- ☐ Sunny
- ☐ Partly Cloudy
- ☐ Cloudy
- ☐ Windy
- ☐ Stormy
- ☐ Light Rain
- ☐ Heavy Rain
- ☐ Light Snow
- ☐ Heavy Snow
- ☐ Other ....

Mood

- ☐ Happy
- ☐ Calm
- ☐ Confident
- ☐ Excited
- ☐ Loving
- ☐ Other
- ☐ Sad
- ☐ Angry
- ☐ Anxious
- ☐ Stressed
- ☐ Self-Critical
- ☐ Tired

Temperature

☐ Hot   ☐ Warm   ☐ Cold   ☐ Damp   ☐ Comfortable

Water

☐ ☐ ☐ ☐ ☐ ☐ ☐ ☐

Energy Level

☆ ☆ ☆ ☆ ☆

Moon

- ☐ New Moon
- ☐ Waxing Crescent
- ☐ First Quarter
- ☐ Waxing Gibbous
- ☐ Full Moon
- ☐ Waning Gibbous
- ☐ Third Quarter
- ☐ Waning Crescent

Bowel Movement

Constipation   *Diarrhea*

Type 1	Type 2	Type 3	Type 4	Type 5	Type 6	Type 7

Medications

Time	Description

Vitamins

Time	Description

Exercise

Time	Intensity	Activity

Breakfast

Lunch

Dinner

Snacks

Menstrual Cycle Symptoms

☐ Cramps ☐ Headache ☐ Backache ☐ Nausea ☐ Fatigue

☐ Tender Breasts ☐ Acne ☐ Bloating ☐ Cravings ☐ Insomnia

☐ Other

Physical Symptoms Log

Period

☐ Spotting ☐ Light ☐ Medium ☐ Heavy

Pain, Discomfort and Skin Changes

(See the Pain Level Reference and/or Glossary for help in describing your symptoms)

Describe your symptoms, pain level and approximate time in the appropriate space below:

☐ Head / Ears / Eyes / Nose / Mouth

☐ Throat / Neck

☐ Shoulders / Arms / Hands

☐ Chest / Heart

☐ Back

☐ Hips / Buttocks / Legs / Feet

☐ Lungs / Breathing (Respiratory)

☐ Stomach / Abdomen (Digestive)

☐ Uterus / Vagina (Reproductive)

☐ Skin

☐ Other

Mark all the places on the diagram below that you are experiencing pain, discomfort, and/or skin changes:

Front

Back

Notes

Daily Wellness Log

Date: ....

S M T W Th F Sa

Weight: ....
Temperature: ....

Hours of Sleep

0 1 2 3 4 5 6 7 8 9 10 11 12+

Sleep Quality

☆ ☆ ☆ ☆ ☆

Weather

- ☐ Sunny ☀
- ☐ Partly Cloudy ☁
- ☐ Cloudy ⛅
- ☐ Windy 🌬
- ☐ Stormy ⛈
- ☐ Light Rain 🌧
- ☐ Heavy Rain 🌧
- ☐ Light Snow 🌨
- ☐ Heavy Snow 🌨
- ☐ Other ....

Mood

- ☐ Happy ☺
- ☐ Calm ☺
- ☐ Confident 😎
- ☐ Excited 😃
- ☐ Loving 😍
- ☐ Other ....
- ☐ Sad ☹
- ☐ Angry 😠
- ☐ Anxious 😰
- ☐ Stressed 😣
- ☐ Self-Critical 😤
- ☐ Tired 😫

Temperature

☐ Hot ☐ Warm ☐ Cold ☐ Damp ☐ Comfortable

Water

🥛 🥛 🥛 🥛 🥛 🥛 🥛 🥛

Energy Level

☆ ☆ ☆ ☆ ☆

Moon

- ☐ New Moon ●
- ☐ Waxing Crescent ●
- ☐ First Quarter ◑
- ☐ Waxing Gibbous ◐
- ☐ Full Moon ○
- ☐ Waning Gibbous ◗
- ☐ Third Quarter ◐
- ☐ Waning Crescent ●

Bowel Movement

Constipation   *Diarrhea*

Type 1	Type 2	Type 3	Type 4	Type 5	Type 6	Type 7

Medications

Time	Description

Vitamins

Time	Description

Exercise

Time	Intensity	Activity

Breakfast

Lunch

Dinner

Snacks

Menstrual Cycle Symptoms

☐ Cramps ☐ Headache ☐ Backache ☐ Nausea ☐ Fatigue

☐ Tender Breasts ☐ Acne ☐ Bloating ☐ Cravings ☐ Insomnia

☐ Other

Physical Symptoms Log

Period

☐ Spotting ☐ Light ☐ Medium ☐ Heavy

Pain, Discomfort and Skin Changes

(See the Pain Level Reference and/or Glossary for help in describing your symptoms)

Describe your symptoms, pain level and approximate time in the appropriate space below:

☐ Head / Ears / Eyes / Nose / Mouth

_____
_____
_____

☐ Throat / Neck

_____
_____
_____

☐ Shoulders / Arms / Hands

_____
_____
_____

☐ Chest / Heart

_____
_____
_____

☐ Back

_____
_____
_____

☐ Hips / Buttocks / Legs / Feet

_____
_____
_____

☐ Lungs / Breathing (Respiratory)

_____
_____
_____

☐ Stomach / Abdomen (Digestive)

_____
_____
_____

☐ Uterus / Vagina (Reproductive)

_____
_____
_____

☐ Skin

_____
_____
_____

☐ Other

_____
_____
_____

Mark all the places on the diagram below that you are experiencing pain, discomfort, and/or skin changes:

Front

Back

Notes

_____
_____
_____
_____

Daily Wellness Log

Date: ....   S M T W Th F Sa

Weight:
Temperature:

Hours of Sleep

0 1 2 3 4 5 6 7 8 9 10 11 12+

Sleep Quality

☆ ☆ ☆ ☆ ☆

Weather

- ☐ Sunny ☀
- ☐ Partly Cloudy ☁
- ☐ Cloudy ⛅
- ☐ Windy 🌬
- ☐ Stormy ⛈
- ☐ Light Rain 🌧
- ☐ Heavy Rain 🌧
- ☐ Light Snow 🌨
- ☐ Heavy Snow 🌨
- ☐ Other ....

Mood

- ☐ Happy 🙂
- ☐ Calm 🙂
- ☐ Confident 😎
- ☐ Excited 😃
- ☐ Loving 😍
- ☐ Other
- ☐ Sad ☹
- ☐ Angry 😣
- ☐ Anxious 😟
- ☐ Stressed 😫
- ☐ Self-Critical 😠
- ☐ Tired 😫

Temperature

☐ Hot   ☐ Warm   ☐ Cold   ☐ Damp   ☐ Comfortable

Water

Energy Level

☆ ☆ ☆ ☆ ☆

Moon

- ☐ New Moon ●
- ☐ Waxing Crescent ◐
- ☐ First Quarter ◑
- ☐ Waxing Gibbous ◑
- ☐ Full Moon ○
- ☐ Waning Gibbous ◑
- ☐ Third Quarter ◐
- ☐ Waning Crescent ◑

Bowel Movement

Constipation   *Diarrhea*

Type 1	Type 2	Type 3	Type 4	Type 5	Type 6	Type 7

Medications

Time	Description

Vitamins

Time	Description

Exercise

Time	Intensity	Activity

Breakfast

Lunch

Dinner

Snacks

Menstrual Cycle Symptoms

- [ ] Cramps
- [ ] Headache
- [ ] Backache
- [ ] Nausea
- [ ] Fatigue
- [ ] Tender Breasts
- [ ] Acne
- [ ] Bloating
- [ ] Cravings
- [ ] Insomnia
- [ ] Other

Physical Symptoms Log

Period

- [ ] Spotting
- [ ] Light
- [ ] Medium
- [ ] Heavy

Pain, Discomfort and Skin Changes

(See the Pain Level Reference and/or Glossary for help in describing your symptoms)

Describe your symptoms, pain level and approximate time in the appropriate space below:

- [ ] Head / Ears / Eyes / Nose / Mouth
  _____
  _____
  _____

- [ ] Throat / Neck
  _____
  _____
  _____

- [ ] Shoulders / Arms / Hands
  _____
  _____
  _____

- [ ] Chest / Heart
  _____
  _____
  _____

- [ ] Back
  _____
  _____
  _____

- [ ] Hips / Buttocks / Legs / Feet
  _____
  _____
  _____

- [ ] Lungs / Breathing (Respiratory)
  _____
  _____
  _____

- [ ] Stomach / Abdomen (Digestive)
  _____
  _____
  _____

- [ ] Uterus / Vagina (Reproductive)
  _____
  _____
  _____

- [ ] Skin
  _____
  _____
  _____

- [ ] Other
  _____
  _____
  _____

Mark all the places on the diagram below that you are experiencing pain, discomfort, and/or skin changes:

Front

Back

Notes

Daily Wellness Log

Date: _____

S M T W Th F Sa

Weight: _____
Temperature: _____

Hours of Sleep

0 1 2 3 4 5 6 7 8 9 10 11 12+

Sleep Quality

☆ ☆ ☆ ☆ ☆

Weather

- [ ] Sunny
- [ ] Partly Cloudy
- [ ] Cloudy
- [ ] Windy
- [ ] Stormy
- [ ] Light Rain
- [ ] Heavy Rain
- [ ] Light Snow
- [ ] Heavy Snow
- [ ] Other

Mood

- [ ] Happy
- [ ] Calm
- [ ] Confident
- [ ] Excited
- [ ] Loving
- [ ] Other
- [ ] Sad
- [ ] Angry
- [ ] Anxious
- [ ] Stressed
- [ ] Self-Critical
- [ ] Tired

Temperature

- [ ] Hot
- [ ] Warm
- [ ] Cold
- [ ] Damp
- [ ] Comfortable

Water

Energy Level

☆ ☆ ☆ ☆ ☆

Moon

- [ ] New Moon
- [ ] Waxing Crescent
- [ ] First Quarter
- [ ] Waxing Gibbous
- [ ] Full Moon
- [ ] Waning Gibbous
- [ ] Third Quarter
- [ ] Waning Crescent

Bowel Movement

Constipation   Diarrhea

Type 1	Type 2	Type 3	Type 4	Type 5	Type 6	Type 7

Medications

Time	Description

Vitamins

Time	Description

Exercise

Time	Intensity	Activity

Breakfast

Lunch

Dinner

Snacks

Menstrual Cycle Symptoms

- [ ] Cramps
- [ ] Headache
- [ ] Backache
- [ ] Nausea
- [ ] Fatigue
- [ ] Tender Breasts
- [ ] Acne
- [ ] Bloating
- [ ] Cravings
- [ ] Insomnia
- [ ] Other

Physical Symptoms Log

Period

- [ ] Spotting
- [ ] Light
- [ ] Medium
- [ ] Heavy

Pain, Discomfort and Skin Changes

(See the Pain Level Reference and/or Glossary for help in describing your symptoms)

Describe your symptoms, pain level and approximate time in the appropriate space below:

- [ ] Head / Ears / Eyes / Nose / Mouth

- [ ] Throat / Neck

- [ ] Shoulders / Arms / Hands

- [ ] Chest / Heart

- [ ] Back

- [ ] Hips / Buttocks / Legs / Feet

- [ ] Lungs / Breathing (Respiratory)

- [ ] Stomach / Abdomen (Digestive)

- [ ] Uterus / Vagina (Reproductive)

- [ ] Skin

- [ ] Other

Mark all the places on the diagram below that you are experiencing pain, discomfort, and/or skin changes:

Front

Back

Notes

Daily Wellness Log

Date: _____

S M T W Th F Sa

Weight: _____
Temperature: _____

Hours of Sleep

0 1 2 3 4 5 6 7 8 9 10 11 12+

Sleep Quality

☆ ☆ ☆ ☆ ☆

Weather

- [ ] Sunny ☀
- [ ] Partly Cloudy ☁
- [ ] Cloudy ⛅
- [ ] Windy 🌬
- [ ] Stormy ⛈
- [ ] Light Rain 🌦
- [ ] Heavy Rain 🌧
- [ ] Light Snow 🌨
- [ ] Heavy Snow ❄
- [ ] Other ....

Mood

- [ ] Happy 🙂
- [ ] Calm 🙂
- [ ] Confident 😎
- [ ] Excited 😃
- [ ] Loving 😍
- [ ] Other
- [ ] Sad 😦
- [ ] Angry 😠
- [ ] Anxious 😕
- [ ] Stressed 😣
- [ ] Self-Critical 😡
- [ ] Tired 😫

Temperature

- [ ] Hot
- [ ] Warm
- [ ] Cold
- [ ] Damp
- [ ] Comfortable

Water

▽ ▽ ▽ ▽ ▽ ▽ ▽ ▽

Energy Level

☆ ☆ ☆ ☆ ☆

Moon

- [ ] New Moon ●
- [ ] Waxing Crescent ◑
- [ ] First Quarter ◐
- [ ] Waxing Gibbous ◑
- [ ] Full Moon ○
- [ ] Waning Gibbous ◔
- [ ] Third Quarter ◑
- [ ] Waning Crescent ◕

Bowel Movement

Constipation   *Diarrhea*

Type 1	Type 2	Type 3	Type 4	Type 5	Type 6	Type 7

Medications

Time	Description

Vitamins

Time	Description

Exercise

Time	Intensity	Activity

Breakfast

Lunch

Dinner

Snacks

Menstrual Cycle Symptoms

- [ ] Cramps
- [ ] Headache
- [ ] Backache
- [ ] Nausea
- [ ] Fatigue
- [ ] Tender Breasts
- [ ] Acne
- [ ] Bloating
- [ ] Cravings
- [ ] Insomnia
- [ ] Other

Physical Symptoms Log

Period

- [ ] Spotting
- [ ] Light
- [ ] Medium
- [ ] Heavy

Pain, Discomfort and Skin Changes

(See the Pain Level Reference and/or Glossary for help in describing your symptoms)

Describe your symptoms, pain level and approximate time in the appropriate space below:

- [ ] Head / Ears / Eyes / Nose / Mouth

- [ ] Throat / Neck

- [ ] Shoulders / Arms / Hands

- [ ] Chest / Heart

- [ ] Back

- [ ] Hips / Buttocks / Legs / Feet

- [ ] Lungs / Breathing (Respiratory)

- [ ] Stomach / Abdomen (Digestive)

- [ ] Uterus / Vagina (Reproductive)

- [ ] Skin

- [ ] Other

Mark all the places on the diagram below that you are experiencing pain, discomfort, and/or skin changes:

Front

Back

Notes

Daily Wellness Log

Date: _____   S M T W Th F Sa

Weight: _____
Temperature: _____

Hours of Sleep

0 1 2 3 4 5 6 7 8 9 10 11 12+

Sleep Quality
☆ ☆ ☆ ☆ ☆

Weather
- [ ] Sunny ☀
- [ ] Partly Cloudy ☁
- [ ] Cloudy ⛅
- [ ] Windy 🌬
- [ ] Stormy ⛈
- [ ] Light Rain 🌦
- [ ] Heavy Rain 🌧
- [ ] Light Snow 🌨
- [ ] Heavy Snow ❄
- [ ] Other ....

Mood
- [ ] Happy 🙂
- [ ] Calm 🙂
- [ ] Confident 😎
- [ ] Excited 😃
- [ ] Loving 😍
- [ ] Other
- [ ] Sad 🙁
- [ ] Angry 😠
- [ ] Anxious 😟
- [ ] Stressed 😣
- [ ] Self-Critical 😡
- [ ] Tired 😫

Temperature
- [ ] Hot
- [ ] Warm
- [ ] Cold
- [ ] Damp
- [ ] Comfortable

Water
▽ ▽ ▽ ▽ ▽ ▽ ▽ ▽

Energy Level
☆ ☆ ☆ ☆ ☆

Moon
- [ ] New Moon ●
- [ ] Waxing Crescent ◑
- [ ] First Quarter ◐
- [ ] Waxing Gibbous ◑
- [ ] Full Moon ○
- [ ] Waning Gibbous ◑
- [ ] Third Quarter ◐
- [ ] Waning Crescent ◑

Bowel Movement

Constipation   *Diarrhea*

Type 1	Type 2	Type 3	Type 4	Type 5	Type 6	Type 7

Medications

Time	Description

Vitamins

Time	Description

Exercise

Time	Intensity	Activity

Breakfast

Lunch

Dinner

Snacks

Menstrual Cycle Symptoms

- [ ] Cramps
- [ ] Headache
- [ ] Backache
- [ ] Nausea
- [ ] Fatigue
- [ ] Tender Breasts
- [ ] Acne
- [ ] Bloating
- [ ] Cravings
- [ ] Insomnia
- [ ] Other

Physical Symptoms Log

Period

- [ ] Spotting
- [ ] Light
- [ ] Medium
- [ ] Heavy

Pain, Discomfort and Skin Changes

(See the Pain Level Reference and/or Glossary for help in describing your symptoms)

Describe your symptoms, pain level and approximate time in the appropriate space below:

- [ ] Head / Ears / Eyes / Nose / Mouth
  _____
  _____
  _____

- [ ] Throat / Neck
  _____
  _____
  _____

- [ ] Shoulders / Arms / Hands
  _____
  _____
  _____

- [ ] Chest / Heart
  _____
  _____
  _____

- [ ] Back
  _____
  _____
  _____

- [ ] Hips / Buttocks / Legs / Feet
  _____
  _____
  _____

- [ ] Lungs / Breathing (Respiratory)
  _____
  _____
  _____

- [ ] Stomach / Abdomen (Digestive)
  _____
  _____
  _____

- [ ] Uterus / Vagina (Reproductive)
  _____
  _____
  _____

- [ ] Skin
  _____
  _____
  _____

- [ ] Other
  _____
  _____
  _____

Mark all the places on the diagram below that you are experiencing pain, discomfort, and/or skin changes:

Front

Back

Notes
_____
_____
_____
_____

Daily Wellness Log

Date: _____

S M T W Th F Sa

Weight: _____
Temperature: _____

Hours of Sleep

0 1 2 3 4 5 6 7 8 9 10 11 12+

Sleep Quality

☆ ☆ ☆ ☆ ☆

Weather

- [ ] Sunny ☀
- [ ] Partly Cloudy ☁
- [ ] Cloudy ⛅
- [ ] Windy 🌬
- [ ] Stormy ⛈
- [ ] Light Rain 🌧
- [ ] Heavy Rain 🌧
- [ ] Light Snow 🌨
- [ ] Heavy Snow 🌨
- [ ] Other _____

Mood

- [ ] Happy ☺
- [ ] Calm ☺
- [ ] Confident 😎
- [ ] Excited 😀
- [ ] Loving 😍
- [ ] Other
- [ ] Sad ☹
- [ ] Angry 😠
- [ ] Anxious 😰
- [ ] Stressed 😖
- [ ] Self-Critical 😣
- [ ] Tired 😫

Temperature

- [ ] Hot
- [ ] Warm
- [ ] Cold
- [ ] Damp
- [ ] Comfortable

Water

🥛 🥛 🥛 🥛 🥛 🥛 🥛 🥛

Energy Level

☆ ☆ ☆ ☆ ☆

Moon

- [ ] New Moon ●
- [ ] Waxing Crescent ●
- [ ] First Quarter ◑
- [ ] Waxing Gibbous ◐
- [ ] Full Moon ○
- [ ] Waning Gibbous ◑
- [ ] Third Quarter ◐
- [ ] Waning Crescent ●

Bowel Movement

Constipation   *Diarrhea*

Type 1	Type 2	Type 3	Type 4	Type 5	Type 6	Type 7

Medications

Time	Description

Vitamins

Time	Description

Exercise

Time	Intensity	Activity

Breakfast

Lunch

Dinner

Snacks

Menstrual Cycle Symptoms

- [ ] Cramps
- [ ] Headache
- [ ] Backache
- [ ] Nausea
- [ ] Fatigue
- [ ] Tender Breasts
- [ ] Acne
- [ ] Bloating
- [ ] Cravings
- [ ] Insomnia
- [ ] Other

Physical Symptoms Log

Period

- [ ] Spotting
- [ ] Light
- [ ] Medium
- [ ] Heavy

Pain, Discomfort and Skin Changes

(See the Pain Level Reference and/or Glossary for help in describing your symptoms)

Describe your symptoms, pain level and approximate time in the appropriate space below:

- [ ] Head / Ears / Eyes / Nose / Mouth

_____

- [ ] Throat / Neck

_____

- [ ] Shoulders / Arms / Hands

_____

- [ ] Chest / Heart

_____

- [ ] Back

_____

- [ ] Hips / Buttocks / Legs / Feet

_____

- [ ] Lungs / Breathing (Respiratory)

_____

- [ ] Stomach / Abdomen (Digestive)

_____

- [ ] Uterus / Vagina (Reproductive)

_____

- [ ] Skin

_____

- [ ] Other

_____

Mark all the places on the diagram below that you are experiencing pain, discomfort, and/or skin changes:

Front

Back

Notes

Daily Wellness Log

Date: ....

S M T W Th F Sa

Weight:
Temperature:

Hours of Sleep

0 1 2 3 4 5 6 7 8 9 10 11 12+

Sleep Quality

☆ ☆ ☆ ☆ ☆

Weather

- [ ] Sunny
- [ ] Partly Cloudy
- [ ] Cloudy
- [ ] Windy
- [ ] Stormy
- [ ] Light Rain
- [ ] Heavy Rain
- [ ] Light Snow
- [ ] Heavy Snow
- [ ] Other

Mood

- [ ] Happy
- [ ] Calm
- [ ] Confident
- [ ] Excited
- [ ] Loving
- [ ] Other
- [ ] Sad
- [ ] Angry
- [ ] Anxious
- [ ] Stressed
- [ ] Self-Critical
- [ ] Tired

Temperature

- [ ] Hot
- [ ] Warm
- [ ] Cold
- [ ] Damp
- [ ] Comfortable

Water

Energy Level

☆ ☆ ☆ ☆ ☆

Moon

- [ ] New Moon
- [ ] Waxing Crescent
- [ ] First Quarter
- [ ] Waxing Gibbous
- [ ] Full Moon
- [ ] Waning Gibbous
- [ ] Third Quarter
- [ ] Waning Crescent

Bowel Movement

Constipation   *Diarrhea*

Type 1	Type 2	Type 3	Type 4	Type 5	Type 6	Type 7

Medications

Time	Description

Vitamins

Time	Description

Exercise

Time	Intensity	Activity

Breakfast

Lunch

Dinner

Snacks

Menstrual Cycle Symptoms

☐ Cramps ☐ Headache ☐ Backache ☐ Nausea ☐ Fatigue

☐ Tender Breasts ☐ Acne ☐ Bloating ☐ Cravings ☐ Insomnia

☐ Other ....

Physical Symptoms Log

Period

☐ Spotting ☐ Light ☐ Medium ☐ Heavy

Pain, Discomfort and Skin Changes

(See the Pain Level Reference and/or Glossary for help in describing your symptoms)

Describe your symptoms, pain level and approximate time in the appropriate space below:

Mark all the places on the diagram below that you are experiencing pain, discomfort, and/or skin changes:

☐ Head / Ears / Eyes / Nose / Mouth
_____
_____
_____

☐ Throat / Neck
_____
_____

☐ Shoulders / Arms / Hands
_____
_____
_____

☐ Chest / Heart
_____
_____

☐ Back
_____
_____
_____

☐ Hips / Buttocks / Legs / Feet
_____
_____
_____

Front

☐ Lungs / Breathing (Respiratory)
_____
_____

☐ Stomach / Abdomen (Digestive)
_____
_____

☐ Uterus / Vagina (Reproductive)
_____
_____

☐ Skin
_____
_____

☐ Other
_____
_____

Back

Notes

_____
_____
_____
_____

Daily Wellness Log

Date: ....

S M T W Th F Sa

Weight:
Temperature:

Hours of Sleep

0 1 2 3 4 5 6 7 8 9 10 11 12+

Sleep Quality

☆ ☆ ☆ ☆ ☆

Weather

- [ ] Sunny ☀
- [ ] Partly Cloudy ⛅
- [ ] Cloudy ⛅
- [ ] Windy 🌬
- [ ] Stormy ⛈
- [ ] Light Rain 🌦
- [ ] Heavy Rain 🌧
- [ ] Light Snow 🌨
- [ ] Heavy Snow 🌨
- [ ] Other

Mood

- [ ] Happy 🙂
- [ ] Calm 🙂
- [ ] Confident 😎
- [ ] Excited 😀
- [ ] Loving 😍
- [ ] Other

- [ ] Sad ☹
- [ ] Angry 😠
- [ ] Anxious 😕
- [ ] Stressed 😣
- [ ] Self-Critical 😡
- [ ] Tired 😫

Temperature

- [ ] Hot
- [ ] Warm
- [ ] Cold
- [ ] Damp
- [ ] Comfortable

Water

🥛 🥛 🥛 🥛 🥛 🥛 🥛 🥛

Energy Level

☆ ☆ ☆ ☆ ☆

Moon

- [ ] New Moon ●
- [ ] Waxing Crescent ◑
- [ ] First Quarter ◐
- [ ] Waxing Gibbous ◑
- [ ] Full Moon ○
- [ ] Waning Gibbous ◑
- [ ] Third Quarter ◑
- [ ] Waning Crescent ◐

Bowel Movement

Constipation   *Diarrhea*

Type 1	Type 2	Type 3	Type 4	Type 5	Type 6	Type 7

Medications

Time	Description

Vitamins

Time	Description

Exercise

Time	Intensity	Activity

Breakfast

Lunch

Dinner

Snacks

Menstrual Cycle Symptoms

- [ ] Cramps
- [ ] Headache
- [ ] Backache
- [ ] Nausea
- [ ] Fatigue
- [ ] Tender Breasts
- [ ] Acne
- [ ] Bloating
- [ ] Cravings
- [ ] Insomnia
- [ ] Other

Physical Symptoms Log

Period

- [ ] Spotting
- [ ] Light
- [ ] Medium
- [ ] Heavy

Pain, Discomfort and Skin Changes

(See the Pain Level Reference and/or Glossary for help in describing your symptoms)

Describe your symptoms, pain level and approximate time in the appropriate space below:

- [ ] Head / Ears / Eyes / Nose / Mouth

- [ ] Shoulders / Arms / Hands

- [ ] Back

- [ ] Lungs / Breathing (Respiratory)

- [ ] Uterus / Vagina (Reproductive)

- [ ] Other

- [ ] Throat / Neck

- [ ] Chest / Heart

- [ ] Hips / Buttocks / Legs / Feet

- [ ] Stomach / Abdomen (Digestive)

- [ ] Skin

Mark all the places on the diagram below that you are experiencing pain, discomfort, and/or skin changes:

Front

Back

Notes

Daily Wellness Log

Date: _____ S M T W Th F Sa

Weight: _____
Temperature: _____

Hours of Sleep

0 1 2 3 4 5 6 7 8 9 10 11 12+

Sleep Quality

☆ ☆ ☆ ☆ ☆

Weather

- [ ] Sunny
- [ ] Partly Cloudy
- [ ] Cloudy
- [ ] Windy
- [ ] Stormy
- [ ] Light Rain
- [ ] Heavy Rain
- [ ] Light Snow
- [ ] Heavy Snow
- [ ] Other _____

Mood

- [ ] Happy
- [ ] Calm
- [ ] Confident
- [ ] Excited
- [ ] Loving
- [ ] Other
- [ ] Sad
- [ ] Angry
- [ ] Anxious
- [ ] Stressed
- [ ] Self-Critical
- [ ] Tired

Temperature

- [ ] Hot
- [ ] Warm
- [ ] Cold
- [ ] Damp
- [ ] Comfortable

Water

🥤 🥤 🥤 🥤 🥤 🥤 🥤 🥤

Energy Level

☆ ☆ ☆ ☆ ☆

Moon

- [ ] New Moon ●
- [ ] Waxing Crescent ●
- [ ] First Quarter ◐
- [ ] Waxing Gibbous ◑
- [ ] Full Moon ○
- [ ] Waning Gibbous ◑
- [ ] Third Quarter ◑
- [ ] Waning Crescent ◐

Bowel Movement

Constipation   *Diarrhea*

| Type 1 | Type 2 | Type 3 | Type 4 | Type 5 | Type 6 | Type 7 |

Medications

Time	Description

Vitamins

Time	Description

Exercise

Time	Intensity	Activity

Breakfast

Lunch

Dinner

Snacks

Menstrual Cycle Symptoms

☐ Cramps   ☐ Headache   ☐ Backache   ☐ Nausea   ☐ Fatigue

☐ Tender Breasts   ☐ Acne   ☐ Bloating   ☐ Cravings   ☐ Insomnia

☐ Other

Physical Symptoms Log

Period

☐ Spotting   ☐ Light   ☐ Medium   ☐ Heavy

Pain, Discomfort and Skin Changes

(See the Pain Level Reference and/or Glossary for help in describing your symptoms)

Describe your symptoms, pain level and approximate time in the appropriate space below:

☐ Head / Ears / Eyes / Nose / Mouth
_____
_____
_____

☐ Throat / Neck
_____
_____

☐ Shoulders / Arms / Hands
_____
_____
_____

☐ Chest / Heart
_____
_____

☐ Back
_____
_____
_____

☐ Hips / Buttocks / Legs / Feet
_____
_____
_____

☐ Lungs / Breathing (Respiratory)
_____
_____

☐ Stomach / Abdomen (Digestive)
_____
_____

☐ Uterus / Vagina (Reproductive)
_____
_____

☐ Skin
_____
_____
_____

☐ Other
_____
_____

Mark all the places on the diagram below that you are experiencing pain, discomfort, and/or skin changes:

Front

Back

Notes
_____
_____
_____
_____

Daily Wellness Log

Date: .... S M T W Th F Sa

Weight:

Temperature:

Hours of Sleep

0 1 2 3 4 5 6 7 8 9 10 11 12+

Sleep Quality

☆ ☆ ☆ ☆ ☆

Weather

- [ ] Sunny ☀
- [ ] Partly Cloudy ☁
- [ ] Cloudy ⛅
- [ ] Windy 🌬
- [ ] Stormy ⛈
- [ ] Light Rain 🌧
- [ ] Heavy Rain 🌧
- [ ] Light Snow 🌨
- [ ] Heavy Snow 🌨
- [ ] Other ....

Mood

- [ ] Happy 🙂
- [ ] Calm 🙂
- [ ] Confident 😎
- [ ] Excited 😀
- [ ] Loving 😍
- [ ] Other
- [ ] Sad 🙁
- [ ] Angry 😣
- [ ] Anxious 😕
- [ ] Stressed 😖
- [ ] Self-Critical 😠
- [ ] Tired 😫

Temperature

- [ ] Hot
- [ ] Warm
- [ ] Cold
- [ ] Damp
- [ ] Comfortable

Water

🥤 🥤 🥤 🥤 🥤 🥤 🥤 🥤

Energy Level

☆ ☆ ☆ ☆ ☆

Moon

- [ ] New Moon ●
- [ ] Waxing Crescent ◐
- [ ] First Quarter ◑
- [ ] Waxing Gibbous ◑
- [ ] Full Moon ○
- [ ] Waning Gibbous ◐
- [ ] Third Quarter ◑
- [ ] Waning Crescent ◐

Bowel Movement

Constipation   Diarrhea

Type 1	Type 2	Type 3	Type 4	Type 5	Type 6	Type 7

Medications

Time	Description

Vitamins

Time	Description

Exercise

Time	Intensity	Activity

Breakfast

Lunch

Dinner

Snacks

Menstrual Cycle Symptoms

- ☐ Cramps   ☐ Headache   ☐ Backache   ☐ Nausea   ☐ Fatigue
- ☐ Tender Breasts   ☐ Acne   ☐ Bloating   ☐ Cravings   ☐ Insomnia
- ☐ Other

Physical Symptoms Log

Period

☐ Spotting   ☐ Light   ☐ Medium   ☐ Heavy

Pain, Discomfort and Skin Changes

(See the Pain Level Reference and/or Glossary for help in describing your symptoms)

Describe your symptoms, pain level and approximate time in the appropriate space below:

☐ Head / Ears / Eyes / Nose / Mouth

_____

_____

☐ Shoulders / Arms / Hands

_____

_____

☐ Back

_____

_____

☐ Lungs / Breathing (Respiratory)

_____

_____

☐ Uterus / Vagina (Reproductive)

_____

_____

☐ Other

_____

_____

☐ Throat / Neck

_____

_____

☐ Chest / Heart

_____

_____

☐ Hips / Buttocks / Legs / Feet

_____

_____

☐ Stomach / Abdomen (Digestive)

_____

_____

☐ Skin

_____

_____

Mark all the places on the diagram below that you are experiencing pain, discomfort, and/or skin changes:

Front

Back

Notes

_____

_____

_____

_____

Daily Wellness Log

Date: ....

S M T W Th F Sa

Weight:

Temperature:

Hours of Sleep

0 1 2 3 4 5 6 7 8 9 10 11 12+

Sleep Quality

☆ ☆ ☆ ☆ ☆

Weather

- ☐ Sunny
- ☐ Partly Cloudy
- ☐ Cloudy
- ☐ Windy
- ☐ Stormy
- ☐ Light Rain
- ☐ Heavy Rain
- ☐ Light Snow
- ☐ Heavy Snow
- ☐ Other

Mood

- ☐ Happy ☺
- ☐ Calm ☺
- ☐ Confident 😎
- ☐ Excited 😄
- ☐ Loving 😍
- ☐ Other
- ☐ Sad ☹
- ☐ Angry 😠
- ☐ Anxious 😟
- ☐ Stressed 😖
- ☐ Self-Critical 😡
- ☐ Tired 😣

Temperature

☐ Hot ☐ Warm ☐ Cold ☐ Damp ☐ Comfortable

Water

🥛 🥛 🥛 🥛 🥛 🥛 🥛 🥛

Energy Level

☆ ☆ ☆ ☆ ☆

Moon

- ☐ New Moon ●
- ☐ Waxing Crescent ◗
- ☐ First Quarter ◑
- ☐ Waxing Gibbous ◕
- ☐ Full Moon ○
- ☐ Waning Gibbous ◑
- ☐ Third Quarter ◐
- ☐ Waning Crescent ◖

Bowel Movement

Constipation   *Diarrhea*

Type 1	Type 2	Type 3	Type 4	Type 5	Type 6	Type 7

Medications

Time	Description

Vitamins

Time	Description

Exercise

Time	Intensity	Activity

Breakfast

Lunch

Dinner

Snacks

Menstrual Cycle Symptoms

- [ ] Cramps
- [ ] Headache
- [ ] Backache
- [ ] Nausea
- [ ] Fatigue
- [ ] Tender Breasts
- [ ] Acne
- [ ] Bloating
- [ ] Cravings
- [ ] Insomnia
- [ ] Other

Physical Symptoms Log

Period

- [ ] Spotting
- [ ] Light
- [ ] Medium
- [ ] Heavy

Pain, Discomfort and Skin Changes

(See the Pain Level Reference and/or Glossary for help in describing your symptoms)

Describe your symptoms, pain level and approximate time in the appropriate space below:

- [ ] Head / Ears / Eyes / Nose / Mouth
  _____
  _____
  _____

- [ ] Throat / Neck
  _____
  _____

- [ ] Shoulders / Arms / Hands
  _____
  _____

- [ ] Chest / Heart
  _____
  _____

- [ ] Back
  _____
  _____

- [ ] Hips / Buttocks / Legs / Feet
  _____
  _____

- [ ] Lungs / Breathing (Respiratory)
  _____
  _____

- [ ] Stomach / Abdomen (Digestive)
  _____
  _____

- [ ] Uterus / Vagina (Reproductive)
  _____
  _____

- [ ] Skin
  _____
  _____

- [ ] Other
  _____
  _____

Mark all the places on the diagram below that you are experiencing pain, discomfort, and/or skin changes:

Front

Back

Notes
_____
_____
_____
_____

Daily Wellness Log

Date: ....

S M T W Th F Sa

Weight: ....
Temperature: ....

Hours of Sleep

0 1 2 3 4 5 6 7 8 9 10 11 12+

Sleep Quality

☆ ☆ ☆ ☆ ☆

Weather

- [ ] Sunny ☀
- [ ] Partly Cloudy ⛅
- [ ] Cloudy ⛅
- [ ] Windy 🌬
- [ ] Stormy ⛈
- [ ] Light Rain 🌦
- [ ] Heavy Rain 🌧
- [ ] Light Snow 🌨
- [ ] Heavy Snow 🌨
- [ ] Other ....

Mood

- [ ] Happy 🙂
- [ ] Calm 🙂
- [ ] Confident 😎
- [ ] Excited 😄
- [ ] Loving 😍
- [ ] Other
- [ ] Sad 🙁
- [ ] Angry 😠
- [ ] Anxious 😫
- [ ] Stressed 😣
- [ ] Self-Critical 😤
- [ ] Tired 😩

Temperature

- [ ] Hot
- [ ] Warm
- [ ] Cold
- [ ] Damp
- [ ] Comfortable

Water

⎕ ⎕ ⎕ ⎕ ⎕ ⎕ ⎕ ⎕

Energy Level

☆ ☆ ☆ ☆ ☆

Moon

- [ ] New Moon ●
- [ ] Waxing Crescent ◗
- [ ] First Quarter ◐
- [ ] Waxing Gibbous ◑
- [ ] Full Moon ○
- [ ] Waning Gibbous ◔
- [ ] Third Quarter ◑
- [ ] Waning Crescent ◖

Bowel Movement

Constipation   *Diarrhea*

Type 1	Type 2	Type 3	Type 4	Type 5	Type 6	Type 7

Medications

Time	Description

Vitamins

Time	Description

Exercise

Time	Intensity	Activity

Breakfast

Lunch

Dinner

Snacks

Menstrual Cycle Symptoms

- [ ] Cramps
- [ ] Headache
- [ ] Backache
- [ ] Nausea
- [ ] Fatigue
- [ ] Tender Breasts
- [ ] Acne
- [ ] Bloating
- [ ] Cravings
- [ ] Insomnia
- [ ] Other

Physical Symptoms Log

Period

- [ ] Spotting
- [ ] Light
- [ ] Medium
- [ ] Heavy

Pain, Discomfort and Skin Changes

(See the Pain Level Reference and/or Glossary for help in describing your symptoms)

Describe your symptoms, pain level and approximate time in the appropriate space below:

- [ ] Head / Ears / Eyes / Nose / Mouth
- [ ] Throat / Neck
- [ ] Shoulders / Arms / Hands
- [ ] Chest / Heart
- [ ] Back
- [ ] Hips / Buttocks / Legs / Feet
- [ ] Lungs / Breathing (Respiratory)
- [ ] Stomach / Abdomen (Digestive)
- [ ] Uterus / Vagina (Reproductive)
- [ ] Skin
- [ ] Other

Mark all the places on the diagram below that you are experiencing pain, discomfort, and/or skin changes:

Front

Back

Notes

Daily Wellness Log

Date: .... S M T W Th F Sa

Weight: ....
Temperature: ....

Hours of Sleep

0 1 2 3 4 5 6 7 8 9 10 11 12+

Sleep Quality

☆ ☆ ☆ ☆ ☆

Weather

- [ ] Sunny ☀
- [ ] Partly Cloudy ☁
- [ ] Cloudy ⛅
- [ ] Windy 🌬
- [ ] Stormy ⛈
- [ ] Light Rain 🌦
- [ ] Heavy Rain 🌧
- [ ] Light Snow 🌨
- [ ] Heavy Snow 🌨
- [ ] Other ....

Mood

- [ ] Happy
- [ ] Calm
- [ ] Confident
- [ ] Excited
- [ ] Loving
- [ ] Other
- [ ] Sad
- [ ] Angry
- [ ] Anxious
- [ ] Stressed
- [ ] Self-Critical
- [ ] Tired

Temperature

- [ ] Hot
- [ ] Warm
- [ ] Cold
- [ ] Damp
- [ ] Comfortable

Water

🥛 🥛 🥛 🥛 🥛 🥛 🥛 🥛

Energy Level

☆ ☆ ☆ ☆ ☆

Moon

- [ ] New Moon ●
- [ ] Waxing Crescent ◗
- [ ] First Quarter ◐
- [ ] Waxing Gibbous ◑
- [ ] Full Moon ○
- [ ] Waning Gibbous ◖
- [ ] Third Quarter ◑
- [ ] Waning Crescent ◐

Bowel Movement

Constipation   *Diarrhea*

Type 1	Type 2	Type 3	Type 4	Type 5	Type 6	Type 7

Medications

Time	Description

Vitamins

Time	Description

Exercise

Time	Intensity	Activity

Breakfast

Lunch

Dinner

Snacks

Menstrual Cycle Symptoms

- [ ] Cramps
- [ ] Headache
- [ ] Backache
- [ ] Nausea
- [ ] Fatigue
- [ ] Tender Breasts
- [ ] Acne
- [ ] Bloating
- [ ] Cravings
- [ ] Insomnia
- [ ] Other _____

Physical Symptoms Log

Period

- [ ] Spotting
- [ ] Light
- [ ] Medium
- [ ] Heavy

Pain, Discomfort and Skin Changes

(See the Pain Level Reference and/or Glossary for help in describing your symptoms)

Describe your symptoms, pain level and approximate time in the appropriate space below:

- [ ] Head / Ears / Eyes / Nose / Mouth
_____
_____
_____

- [ ] Throat / Neck
_____
_____

- [ ] Shoulders / Arms / Hands
_____
_____

- [ ] Chest / Heart
_____
_____

- [ ] Back
_____
_____

- [ ] Hips / Buttocks / Legs / Feet
_____
_____

- [ ] Lungs / Breathing (Respiratory)
_____
_____

- [ ] Stomach / Abdomen (Digestive)
_____
_____

- [ ] Uterus / Vagina (Reproductive)
_____
_____

- [ ] Skin
_____
_____

- [ ] Other
_____
_____

Mark all the places on the diagram below that you are experiencing pain, discomfort, and/or skin changes:

Front

Back

Notes
_____
_____
_____
_____
_____

Daily Wellness Log

Date: ....   S   M   T   W   Th   F   Sa

Weight:
Temperature:

Hours of Sleep

0   1   2   3   4   5   6   7   8   9   10   11   12+

Sleep Quality

☆ ☆ ☆ ☆ ☆

Weather

- ☐ Sunny
- ☐ Partly Cloudy
- ☐ Cloudy
- ☐ Windy
- ☐ Stormy
- ☐ Light Rain
- ☐ Heavy Rain
- ☐ Light Snow
- ☐ Heavy Snow
- ☐ Other ....

Mood

- ☐ Happy
- ☐ Calm
- ☐ Confident
- ☐ Excited
- ☐ Loving
- ☐ Other ....
- ☐ Sad
- ☐ Angry
- ☐ Anxious
- ☐ Stressed
- ☐ Self-Critical
- ☐ Tired

Temperature

☐ Hot   ☐ Warm   ☐ Cold   ☐ Damp   ☐ Comfortable

Water

Energy Level

☆ ☆ ☆ ☆ ☆

Moon

- ☐ New Moon
- ☐ Waxing Crescent
- ☐ First Quarter
- ☐ Waxing Gibbous
- ☐ Full Moon
- ☐ Waning Gibbous
- ☐ Third Quarter
- ☐ Waning Crescent

Bowel Movement

Constipation   *Diarrhea*

Type 1	Type 2	Type 3	Type 4	Type 5	Type 6	Type 7

Medications

Time	Description

Vitamins

Time	Description

Exercise

Time	Intensity	Activity

Breakfast

Lunch

Dinner

Snacks

Menstrual Cycle Symptoms

- [ ] Cramps
- [ ] Headache
- [ ] Backache
- [ ] Nausea
- [ ] Fatigue
- [ ] Tender Breasts
- [ ] Acne
- [ ] Bloating
- [ ] Cravings
- [ ] Insomnia
- [ ] Other

Physical Symptoms Log

Period

- [ ] Spotting
- [ ] Light
- [ ] Medium
- [ ] Heavy

Pain, Discomfort and Skin Changes

(See the Pain Level Reference and/or Glossary for help in describing your symptoms)

Describe your symptoms, pain level and approximate time in the appropriate space below:

- [ ] Head / Ears / Eyes / Nose / Mouth

- [ ] Throat / Neck

- [ ] Shoulders / Arms / Hands

- [ ] Chest / Heart

- [ ] Back

- [ ] Hips / Buttocks / Legs / Feet

- [ ] Lungs / Breathing (Respiratory)

- [ ] Stomach / Abdomen (Digestive)

- [ ] Uterus / Vagina (Reproductive)

- [ ] Skin

- [ ] Other

Mark all the places on the diagram below that you are experiencing pain, discomfort, and/or skin changes:

Front

Back

Notes

Daily Wellness Log

Date: ....

S M T W Th F Sa

Weight:
Temperature:

Hours of Sleep

0 1 2 3 4 5 6 7 8 9 10 11 12+

Sleep Quality

☆ ☆ ☆ ☆ ☆

Weather

- ☐ Sunny ☀
- ☐ Partly Cloudy ☁
- ☐ Cloudy ⛅
- ☐ Windy 🌬
- ☐ Stormy ⛈
- ☐ Light Rain 🌦
- ☐ Heavy Rain 🌧
- ☐ Light Snow 🌨
- ☐ Heavy Snow ❄
- ☐ Other ....

Mood

- ☐ Happy 🙂
- ☐ Calm 🙂
- ☐ Confident 😎
- ☐ Excited 😃
- ☐ Loving 😍
- ☐ Other ....
- ☐ Sad ☹
- ☐ Angry 😠
- ☐ Anxious 😣
- ☐ Stressed 😖
- ☐ Self-Critical 😤
- ☐ Tired 😫

Temperature

- ☐ Hot
- ☐ Warm
- ☐ Cold
- ☐ Damp
- ☐ Comfortable

Water

🥤 🥤 🥤 🥤 🥤 🥤 🥤 🥤

Energy Level

☆ ☆ ☆ ☆ ☆

Moon

- ☐ New Moon ●
- ☐ Waxing Crescent ◗
- ☐ First Quarter ◑
- ☐ Waxing Gibbous ◒
- ☐ Full Moon ○
- ☐ Waning Gibbous ◔
- ☐ Third Quarter ◐
- ☐ Waning Crescent ◖

Bowel Movement

Constipation   *Diarrhea*

Type 1	Type 2	Type 3	Type 4	Type 5	Type 6	Type 7

Medications

Time	Description

Vitamins

Time	Description

Exercise

Time	Intensity	Activity

Breakfast

Lunch

Dinner

Snacks

Menstrual Cycle Symptoms

- [ ] Cramps
- [ ] Headache
- [ ] Backache
- [ ] Nausea
- [ ] Fatigue
- [ ] Tender Breasts
- [ ] Acne
- [ ] Bloating
- [ ] Cravings
- [ ] Insomnia
- [ ] Other

Physical Symptoms Log

Period

- [ ] Spotting
- [ ] Light
- [ ] Medium
- [ ] Heavy

Pain, Discomfort and Skin Changes

(See the Pain Level Reference and/or Glossary for help in describing your symptoms)

Describe your symptoms, pain level and approximate time in the appropriate space below:

- [ ] Head / Ears / Eyes / Nose / Mouth

- [ ] Throat / Neck

- [ ] Shoulders / Arms / Hands

- [ ] Chest / Heart

- [ ] Back

- [ ] Hips / Buttocks / Legs / Feet

- [ ] Lungs / Breathing (Respiratory)

- [ ] Stomach / Abdomen (Digestive)

- [ ] Uterus / Vagina (Reproductive)

- [ ] Skin

- [ ] Other

Mark all the places on the diagram below that you are experiencing pain, discomfort, and/or skin changes:

Front

Back

Notes

Daily Wellness Log

Date: _____   S M T W Th F Sa

Weight: _____
Temperature: _____

Hours of Sleep

0 1 2 3 4 5 6 7 8 9 10 11 12+

Sleep Quality

☆ ☆ ☆ ☆ ☆

Weather

- ☐ Sunny ☀
- ☐ Partly Cloudy ☁
- ☐ Cloudy ⛅
- ☐ Windy 🌬
- ☐ Stormy ⛈
- ☐ Light Rain 🌦
- ☐ Heavy Rain 🌧
- ☐ Light Snow 🌨
- ☐ Heavy Snow ❄
- ☐ Other _____

Mood

- ☐ Happy 🙂
- ☐ Calm 🙂
- ☐ Confident 😎
- ☐ Excited 😃
- ☐ Loving 😍
- ☐ Other
- ☐ Sad ☹
- ☐ Angry 😠
- ☐ Anxious 😬
- ☐ Stressed 😫
- ☐ Self-Critical 😤
- ☐ Tired 😩

Temperature

☐ Hot   ☐ Warm   ☐ Cold   ☐ Damp   ☐ Comfortable

Water

🥤 🥤 🥤 🥤 🥤 🥤 🥤 🥤

Energy Level

☆ ☆ ☆ ☆ ☆

Moon

- ☐ New Moon ●
- ☐ Waxing Crescent ◕
- ☐ First Quarter ◑
- ☐ Waxing Gibbous ◑
- ☐ Full Moon ○
- ☐ Waning Gibbous ◔
- ☐ Third Quarter ◐
- ☐ Waning Crescent ◖

Bowel Movement

Constipation   *Diarrhea*

Type 1	Type 2	Type 3	Type 4	Type 5	Type 6	Type 7

Medications

Time	Description

Vitamins

Time	Description

Exercise

Time	Intensity	Activity

Breakfast

Lunch

Dinner

Snacks

Menstrual Cycle Symptoms

- [ ] Cramps
- [ ] Headache
- [ ] Backache
- [ ] Nausea
- [ ] Fatigue
- [ ] Tender Breasts
- [ ] Acne
- [ ] Bloating
- [ ] Cravings
- [ ] Insomnia
- [ ] Other

Physical Symptoms Log

Period

- [ ] Spotting
- [ ] Light
- [ ] Medium
- [ ] Heavy

Pain, Discomfort and Skin Changes

(See the Pain Level Reference and/or Glossary for help in describing your symptoms)

Describe your symptoms, pain level and approximate time in the appropriate space below:

- [ ] Head / Ears / Eyes / Nose / Mouth
  _____
  _____
  _____

- [ ] Throat / Neck
  _____
  _____
  _____

- [ ] Shoulders / Arms / Hands
  _____
  _____

- [ ] Chest / Heart
  _____
  _____

- [ ] Back
  _____
  _____

- [ ] Hips / Buttocks / Legs / Feet
  _____
  _____

- [ ] Lungs / Breathing (Respiratory)
  _____
  _____

- [ ] Stomach / Abdomen (Digestive)
  _____
  _____

- [ ] Uterus / Vagina (Reproductive)
  _____
  _____

- [ ] Skin
  _____
  _____

- [ ] Other
  _____
  _____

Mark all the places on the diagram below that you are experiencing pain, discomfort, and/or skin changes:

Front

Back

Notes
_____
_____
_____
_____

Daily Wellness Log

Date: ....   S M T W Th F Sa

Weight:
Temperature:

Hours of Sleep

0 1 2 3 4 5 6 7 8 9 10 11 12+

Sleep Quality

☆ ☆ ☆ ☆ ☆

Weather

- [ ] Sunny ☀
- [ ] Partly Cloudy ☁
- [ ] Cloudy ⛅
- [ ] Windy 🌬
- [ ] Stormy ⛈
- [ ] Light Rain 🌧
- [ ] Heavy Rain 🌧
- [ ] Light Snow 🌨
- [ ] Heavy Snow 🌨
- [ ] Other ....

Mood

- [ ] Happy ☺
- [ ] Calm ☺
- [ ] Confident 😎
- [ ] Excited 😊
- [ ] Loving 😍
- [ ] Other
- [ ] Sad ☹
- [ ] Angry 😠
- [ ] Anxious 😕
- [ ] Stressed 😣
- [ ] Self-Critical 😡
- [ ] Tired 😫

Temperature

- [ ] Hot
- [ ] Warm
- [ ] Cold
- [ ] Damp
- [ ] Comfortable

Water

⊔ ⊔ ⊔ ⊔ ⊔ ⊔ ⊔ ⊔

Energy Level

☆ ☆ ☆ ☆ ☆

Moon

- [ ] New Moon ●
- [ ] Waxing Crescent ●
- [ ] First Quarter ◑
- [ ] Waxing Gibbous ◑
- [ ] Full Moon ○
- [ ] Waning Gibbous ◐
- [ ] Third Quarter ◐
- [ ] Waning Crescent ●

Bowel Movement

Constipation   *Diarrhea*

Type 1	Type 2	Type 3	Type 4	Type 5	Type 6	Type 7

Medications

Time	Description

Vitamins

Time	Description

Exercise

Time	Intensity	Activity

Breakfast

Lunch

Dinner

Snacks

Menstrual Cycle Symptoms

☐ Cramps ☐ Headache ☐ Backache ☐ Nausea ☐ Fatigue

☐ Tender Breasts ☐ Acne ☐ Bloating ☐ Cravings ☐ Insomnia

☐ Other

Physical Symptoms Log

Period

☐ Spotting ☐ Light ☐ Medium ☐ Heavy

Pain, Discomfort and Skin Changes

(See the Pain Level Reference and/or Glossary for help in describing your symptoms)

Describe your symptoms, pain level and approximate time in the appropriate space below:

Mark all the places on the diagram below that you are experiencing pain, discomfort, and/or skin changes:

☐ Head / Ears / Eyes / Nose / Mouth

☐ Throat / Neck

☐ Shoulders / Arms / Hands

☐ Chest / Heart

☐ Back

☐ Hips / Buttocks / Legs / Feet

☐ Lungs / Breathing (Respiratory)

☐ Stomach / Abdomen (Digestive)

☐ Uterus / Vagina (Reproductive)

☐ Skin

☐ Other

Front

Back

Notes

Daily Wellness Log

Date: _____   S M T W Th F Sa

Weight: _____

Temperature: _____

Hours of Sleep

0 1 2 3 4 5 6 7 8 9 10 11 12+

Sleep Quality

☆ ☆ ☆ ☆ ☆

Weather

- [ ] Sunny ☀
- [ ] Partly Cloudy ☁
- [ ] Cloudy ⛅
- [ ] Windy
- [ ] Stormy ⛈
- [ ] Light Rain 🌧
- [ ] Heavy Rain 🌧
- [ ] Light Snow 🌨
- [ ] Heavy Snow 🌨
- [ ] Other _____

Mood

- [ ] Happy ☺
- [ ] Calm ☺
- [ ] Confident 😎
- [ ] Excited ☺
- [ ] Loving 😍
- [ ] Other _____
- [ ] Sad ☹
- [ ] Angry 😠
- [ ] Anxious 😣
- [ ] Stressed 😣
- [ ] Self-Critical 😡
- [ ] Tired 😫

Temperature

- [ ] Hot
- [ ] Warm
- [ ] Cold
- [ ] Damp
- [ ] Comfortable

Water

🥛 🥛 🥛 🥛 🥛 🥛 🥛 🥛

Energy Level

☆ ☆ ☆ ☆ ☆

Moon

- [ ] New Moon ●
- [ ] Waxing Crescent ●
- [ ] First Quarter ◐
- [ ] Waxing Gibbous ◐
- [ ] Full Moon ○
- [ ] Waning Gibbous ◑
- [ ] Third Quarter ◑
- [ ] Waning Crescent ◐

Bowel Movement

Constipation   *Diarrhea*

Type 1	Type 2	Type 3	Type 4	Type 5	Type 6	Type 7

Medications

Time	Description

Vitamins

Time	Description

Exercise

Time	Intensity	Activity

Breakfast

Lunch

Dinner

Snacks

Menstrual Cycle Symptoms

- [ ] Cramps
- [ ] Headache
- [ ] Backache
- [ ] Nausea
- [ ] Fatigue
- [ ] Tender Breasts
- [ ] Acne
- [ ] Bloating
- [ ] Cravings
- [ ] Insomnia
- [ ] Other

Physical Symptoms Log

Period

- [ ] Spotting
- [ ] Light
- [ ] Medium
- [ ] Heavy

Pain, Discomfort and Skin Changes

(See the Pain Level Reference and/or Glossary for help in describing your symptoms)

Describe your symptoms, pain level and approximate time in the appropriate space below:

- [ ] Head / Ears / Eyes / Nose / Mouth

- [ ] Throat / Neck

- [ ] Shoulders / Arms / Hands

- [ ] Chest / Heart

- [ ] Back

- [ ] Hips / Buttocks / Legs / Feet

- [ ] Lungs / Breathing (Respiratory)

- [ ] Stomach / Abdomen (Digestive)

- [ ] Uterus / Vagina (Reproductive)

- [ ] Skin

- [ ] Other

Mark all the places on the diagram below that you are experiencing pain, discomfort, and/or skin changes:

Front

Back

Notes

Daily Wellness Log

Date: ....   S M T W Th F Sa

Weight:

Temperature:

Hours of Sleep

0 1 2 3 4 5 6 7 8 9 10 11 12+

Sleep Quality

☆ ☆ ☆ ☆ ☆

Weather

- [ ] Sunny ☀
- [ ] Partly Cloudy ☁
- [ ] Cloudy ⛅
- [ ] Windy 🌬
- [ ] Stormy ⛈
- [ ] Light Rain 🌦
- [ ] Heavy Rain 🌧
- [ ] Light Snow 🌨
- [ ] Heavy Snow 🌨
- [ ] Other ....

Mood

- [ ] Happy ☺
- [ ] Calm ☺
- [ ] Confident 😎
- [ ] Excited 😃
- [ ] Loving 😍
- [ ] Other
- [ ] Sad ☹
- [ ] Angry 😠
- [ ] Anxious 😰
- [ ] Stressed 😣
- [ ] Self-Critical 😤
- [ ] Tired 😫

Temperature

- [ ] Hot
- [ ] Warm
- [ ] Cold
- [ ] Damp
- [ ] Comfortable

Water

⊔ ⊔ ⊔ ⊔ ⊔ ⊔ ⊔ ⊔

Energy Level

☆ ☆ ☆ ☆ ☆

Moon

- [ ] New Moon ●
- [ ] Waxing Crescent ●
- [ ] First Quarter ◑
- [ ] Waxing Gibbous ◑
- [ ] Full Moon ○
- [ ] Waning Gibbous ◐
- [ ] Third Quarter ◐
- [ ] Waning Crescent ◑

Bowel Movement

Constipation   *Diarrhea*

Type 1	Type 2	Type 3	Type 4	Type 5	Type 6	Type 7

Medications

Time	Description

Vitamins

Time	Description

Exercise

Time	Intensity	Activity

Breakfast

Lunch

Dinner

Snacks

Menstrual Cycle Symptoms

- ☐ Cramps ☐ Headache ☐ Backache ☐ Nausea ☐ Fatigue
- ☐ Tender Breasts ☐ Acne ☐ Bloating ☐ Cravings ☐ Insomnia
- ☐ Other

Physical Symptoms Log

Period

☐ Spotting ☐ Light ☐ Medium ☐ Heavy

Pain, Discomfort and Skin Changes

(See the Pain Level Reference and/or Glossary for help in describing your symptoms)

Describe your symptoms, pain level and approximate time in the appropriate space below:

☐ Head / Ears / Eyes / Nose / Mouth

_____
_____
_____

☐ Throat / Neck

_____
_____
_____

☐ Shoulders / Arms / Hands

_____
_____
_____

☐ Chest / Heart

_____
_____
_____

☐ Back

_____
_____
_____

☐ Hips / Buttocks / Legs / Feet

_____
_____
_____

☐ Lungs / Breathing (Respiratory)

_____
_____

☐ Stomach / Abdomen (Digestive)

_____
_____

☐ Uterus / Vagina (Reproductive)

_____
_____
_____

☐ Skin

_____
_____
_____

☐ Other

_____
_____

Mark all the places on the diagram below that you are experiencing pain, discomfort, and/or skin changes:

Front

Back

Notes

Daily Wellness Log

Date: _____   S M T W Th F Sa

Weight: _____
Temperature: _____

Hours of Sleep

0 1 2 3 4 5 6 7 8 9 10 11 12+

Sleep Quality

☆ ☆ ☆ ☆ ☆

Weather

- [ ] Sunny ☀
- [ ] Partly Cloudy ☁
- [ ] Cloudy ⛅
- [ ] Windy 🌬
- [ ] Stormy ⛈
- [ ] Light Rain 🌦
- [ ] Heavy Rain 🌧
- [ ] Light Snow 🌨
- [ ] Heavy Snow 🌨
- [ ] Other _____

Temperature

- [ ] Hot
- [ ] Warm
- [ ] Cold
- [ ] Damp
- [ ] Comfortable

Moon

- [ ] New Moon ●
- [ ] Waxing Crescent ●
- [ ] First Quarter ◐
- [ ] Waxing Gibbous ◐
- [ ] Full Moon ○
- [ ] Waning Gibbous ◐
- [ ] Third Quarter ◑
- [ ] Waning Crescent ◕

Mood

- [ ] Happy 🙂
- [ ] Calm 🙂
- [ ] Confident 😎
- [ ] Excited 😃
- [ ] Loving 😍
- [ ] Other
- [ ] Sad ☹
- [ ] Angry 😠
- [ ] Anxious 😦
- [ ] Stressed 😖
- [ ] Self-Critical 😠
- [ ] Tired 😫

Water

⊔ ⊔ ⊔ ⊔ ⊔ ⊔ ⊔ ⊔

Energy Level

☆ ☆ ☆ ☆ ☆

Bowel Movement

Constipation   *Diarrhea*

Type 1	Type 2	Type 3	Type 4	Type 5	Type 6	Type 7

Medications

Time	Description

Vitamins

Time	Description

Exercise

Time	Intensity	Activity

Breakfast

Lunch

Dinner

Snacks

Menstrual Cycle Symptoms

- [ ] Cramps
- [ ] Headache
- [ ] Backache
- [ ] Nausea
- [ ] Fatigue
- [ ] Tender Breasts
- [ ] Acne
- [ ] Bloating
- [ ] Cravings
- [ ] Insomnia
- [ ] Other

Physical Symptoms Log

Period

- [ ] Spotting
- [ ] Light
- [ ] Medium
- [ ] Heavy

Pain, Discomfort and Skin Changes

(See the Pain Level Reference and/or Glossary for help in describing your symptoms)

Describe your symptoms, pain level and approximate time in the appropriate space below:

- [ ] Head / Ears / Eyes / Nose / Mouth
- [ ] Throat / Neck
- [ ] Shoulders / Arms / Hands
- [ ] Chest / Heart
- [ ] Back
- [ ] Hips / Buttocks / Legs / Feet
- [ ] Lungs / Breathing (Respiratory)
- [ ] Stomach / Abdomen (Digestive)
- [ ] Uterus / Vagina (Reproductive)
- [ ] Skin
- [ ] Other

Mark all the places on the diagram below that you are experiencing pain, discomfort, and/or skin changes:

Front

Back

Notes

Daily Wellness Log

Date: ....

S   M   T   W   Th   F   Sa

Weight:
Temperature:

Hours of Sleep

0   1   2   3   4   5   6   7   8   9   10   11   12+

Sleep Quality

☆ ☆ ☆ ☆ ☆

Weather

- [ ] Sunny ☀
- [ ] Partly Cloudy ☁
- [ ] Cloudy ⛅
- [ ] Windy 🌬
- [ ] Stormy ⛈
- [ ] Light Rain 🌧
- [ ] Heavy Rain 🌧
- [ ] Light Snow 🌨
- [ ] Heavy Snow 🌨
- [ ] Other ....

Mood

- [ ] Happy ☺
- [ ] Calm ☺
- [ ] Confident 😎
- [ ] Excited ☺
- [ ] Loving 😍
- [ ] Other ....
- [ ] Sad ☹
- [ ] Angry 😠
- [ ] Anxious 😣
- [ ] Stressed 😖
- [ ] Self-Critical 😠
- [ ] Tired 😫

Temperature

- [ ] Hot
- [ ] Warm
- [ ] Cold
- [ ] Damp
- [ ] Comfortable

Water

⊔ ⊔ ⊔ ⊔ ⊔ ⊔ ⊔ ⊔

Energy Level

☆ ☆ ☆ ☆ ☆

Moon

- [ ] New Moon ●
- [ ] Waxing Crescent ◐
- [ ] First Quarter ◑
- [ ] Waxing Gibbous ◑
- [ ] Full Moon ○
- [ ] Waning Gibbous ◑
- [ ] Third Quarter ◐
- [ ] Waning Crescent ◐

Bowel Movement

Constipation   *Diarrhea*

Type 1	Type 2	Type 3	Type 4	Type 5	Type 6	Type 7

Medications

Time	Description

Vitamins

Time	Description

Exercise

Time	Intensity	Activity

Breakfast

Lunch

Dinner

Snacks

Menstrual Cycle Symptoms

☐ Cramps ☐ Headache ☐ Backache ☐ Nausea ☐ Fatigue

☐ Tender Breasts ☐ Acne ☐ Bloating ☐ Cravings ☐ Insomnia

☐ Other

Physical Symptoms Log

Period

☐ Spotting ☐ Light ☐ Medium ☐ Heavy

Pain, Discomfort and Skin Changes

(See the Pain Level Reference and/or Glossary for help in describing your symptoms)

Describe your symptoms, pain level and approximate time in the appropriate space below:

☐ Head / Ears / Eyes / Nose / Mouth

☐ Throat / Neck

☐ Shoulders / Arms / Hands

☐ Chest / Heart

☐ Back

☐ Hips / Buttocks / Legs / Feet

☐ Lungs / Breathing (Respiratory)

☐ Stomach / Abdomen (Digestive)

☐ Uterus / Vagina (Reproductive)

☐ Skin

☐ Other

Mark all the places on the diagram below that you are experiencing pain, discomfort, and/or skin changes:

Front

Back

Notes

Daily Wellness Log

Date: ....   S   M   T   W   Th   F   Sa

Weight:
Temperature:

Hours of Sleep

0 1 2 3 4 5 6 7 8 9 10 11 12+

Sleep Quality
☆ ☆ ☆ ☆ ☆

Weather
- [ ] Sunny ☀
- [ ] Partly Cloudy ☁
- [ ] Cloudy ⛅
- [ ] Windy 🌬
- [ ] Stormy ⚡
- [ ] Light Rain 🌦
- [ ] Heavy Rain 🌧
- [ ] Light Snow 🌨
- [ ] Heavy Snow 🌨
- [ ] Other ....

Mood
- [ ] Happy 🙂
- [ ] Calm 🙂
- [ ] Confident 😎
- [ ] Excited 😃
- [ ] Loving 😍
- [ ] Other ....
- [ ] Sad ☹
- [ ] Angry 😠
- [ ] Anxious 😖
- [ ] Stressed 😫
- [ ] Self-Critical 😤
- [ ] Tired 😩

Temperature
- [ ] Hot
- [ ] Warm
- [ ] Cold
- [ ] Damp
- [ ] Comfortable

Water
▽ ▽ ▽ ▽ ▽ ▽ ▽ ▽

Energy Level
☆ ☆ ☆ ☆ ☆

Moon
- [ ] New Moon ●
- [ ] Waxing Crescent ◗
- [ ] First Quarter ◑
- [ ] Waxing Gibbous ◐
- [ ] Full Moon ○
- [ ] Waning Gibbous ◑
- [ ] Third Quarter ◐
- [ ] Waning Crescent ◖

Bowel Movement

Constipation						Diarrhea
Type 1	Type 2	Type 3	Type 4	Type 5	Type 6	Type 7

Medication

Time	Description

Vitamins

Time	Description

Exercise

Time	Intensity	Activity

Breakfast

Lunch

Dinner

Snacks

Menstrual Cycle Symptoms

☐ Cramps ☐ Headache ☐ Backache ☐ Nausea ☐ Fatigue

☐ Tender Breasts ☐ Acne ☐ Bloating ☐ Cravings ☐ Insomnia

☐ Other _____

Physical Symptoms Log

Period

☐ Spotting ☐ Light ☐ Medium ☐ Heavy

Pain, Discomfort and Skin Changes

(See the Pain Level Reference and/or Glossary for help in describing your symptoms)

Describe your symptoms, pain level and approximate time in the appropriate space below:

☐ Head / Ears / Eyes / Nose / Mouth
_____
_____
_____

☐ Shoulders / Arms / Hands
_____
_____
_____

☐ Back
_____
_____
_____

☐ Lungs / Breathing (Respiratory)
_____
_____

☐ Uterus / Vagina (Reproductive)
_____
_____

☐ Other
_____
_____

☐ Throat / Neck
_____
_____
_____

☐ Chest / Heart
_____
_____
_____

☐ Hips / Buttocks / Legs / Feet
_____
_____
_____

☐ Stomach / Abdomen (Digestive)
_____
_____

☐ Skin
_____
_____

Mark all the places on the diagram below that you are experiencing pain, discomfort, and/or skin changes:

Front

Back

Notes
_____
_____
_____
_____
_____

Daily Wellness Log

Date: _____   S M T W Th F Sa

Weight: _____

Temperature: _____

Hours of Sleep

0 1 2 3 4 5 6 7 8 9 10 11 12+

Sleep Quality

☆ ☆ ☆ ☆ ☆

Weather

- [ ] Sunny
- [ ] Partly Cloudy
- [ ] Cloudy
- [ ] Windy
- [ ] Stormy
- [ ] Light Rain
- [ ] Heavy Rain
- [ ] Light Snow
- [ ] Heavy Snow
- [ ] Other _____

Mood

- [ ] Happy
- [ ] Calm
- [ ] Confident
- [ ] Excited
- [ ] Loving
- [ ] Other
- [ ] Sad
- [ ] Angry
- [ ] Anxious
- [ ] Stressed
- [ ] Self-Critical
- [ ] Tired

Temperature

- [ ] Hot
- [ ] Warm
- [ ] Cold
- [ ] Damp
- [ ] Comfortable

Water

Energy Level

☆ ☆ ☆ ☆ ☆

Moon

- [ ] New Moon
- [ ] Waxing Crescent
- [ ] First Quarter
- [ ] Waxing Gibbous
- [ ] Full Moon
- [ ] Waning Gibbous
- [ ] Third Quarter
- [ ] Waning Crescent

Bowel Movement

Constipation   *Diarrhea*

Type 1	Type 2	Type 3	Type 4	Type 5	Type 6	Type 7

Medications

Time	Description

Vitamins

Time	Description

Exercise

Time	Intensity	Activity

Breakfast

Lunch

Dinner

Snacks

Menstrual Cycle Symptoms

☐ Cramps   ☐ Headache   ☐ Backache   ☐ Nausea   ☐ Fatigue

☐ Tender Breasts   ☐ Acne   ☐ Bloating   ☐ Cravings   ☐ Insomnia

☐ Other

Physical Symptoms Log

Period

☐ Spotting   ☐ Light   ☐ Medium   ☐ Heavy

Pain, Discomfort and Skin Changes

(See the Pain Level Reference and/or Glossary for help in describing your symptoms)

Describe your symptoms, pain level and approximate time in the appropriate space below:

☐ Head / Ears / Eyes / Nose / Mouth

☐ Throat / Neck

☐ Shoulders / Arms / Hands

☐ Chest / Heart

☐ Back

☐ Hips / Buttocks / Legs / Feet

☐ Lungs / Breathing (Respiratory)

☐ Stomach / Abdomen (Digestive)

☐ Uterus / Vagina (Reproductive)

☐ Skin

☐ Other

Mark all the places on the diagram below that you are experiencing pain, discomfort, and/or skin changes:

Front

Back

Notes

Daily Wellness Log

Date: _____   S M T W Th F Sa

Weight: _____
Temperature: _____

Hours of Sleep

0 1 2 3 4 5 6 7 8 9 10 11 12+

Sleep Quality

☆ ☆ ☆ ☆ ☆

Weather

- [ ] Sunny
- [ ] Partly Cloudy
- [ ] Cloudy
- [ ] Windy
- [ ] Stormy
- [ ] Light Rain
- [ ] Heavy Rain
- [ ] Light Snow
- [ ] Heavy Snow
- [ ] Other

Mood

- [ ] Happy
- [ ] Calm
- [ ] Confident
- [ ] Excited
- [ ] Loving
- [ ] Other
- [ ] Sad
- [ ] Angry
- [ ] Anxious
- [ ] Stressed
- [ ] Self-Critical
- [ ] Tired

Temperature

- [ ] Hot
- [ ] Warm
- [ ] Cold
- [ ] Damp
- [ ] Comfortable

Water

Energy Level

☆ ☆ ☆ ☆ ☆

Moon

- [ ] New Moon
- [ ] Waxing Crescent
- [ ] First Quarter
- [ ] Waxing Gibbous
- [ ] Full Moon
- [ ] Waning Gibbous
- [ ] Third Quarter
- [ ] Waning Crescent

Bowel Movement

Constipation   *Diarrhea*

Type 1	Type 2	Type 3	Type 4	Type 5	Type 6	Type 7

Medication

Time	Description

Vitamins

Time	Description

Exercise

Time	Intensity	Activity

Breakfast

Lunch

Dinner

Snacks

Menstrual Cycle Symptoms

- [ ] Cramps
- [ ] Headache
- [ ] Backache
- [ ] Nausea
- [ ] Fatigue
- [ ] Tender Breasts
- [ ] Acne
- [ ] Bloating
- [ ] Cravings
- [ ] Insomnia
- [ ] Other

Physical Symptoms Log

Period

- [ ] Spotting
- [ ] Light
- [ ] Medium
- [ ] Heavy

Pain, Discomfort and Skin Changes

(See the Pain Level Reference and/or Glossary for help in describing your symptoms)

Describe your symptoms, pain level and approximate time in the appropriate space below:

- [ ] Head / Ears / Eyes / Nose / Mouth

- [ ] Throat / Neck

- [ ] Shoulders / Arms / Hands

- [ ] Chest / Heart

- [ ] Back

- [ ] Hips / Buttocks / Legs / Feet

- [ ] Lungs / Breathing (Respiratory)

- [ ] Stomach / Abdomen (Digestive)

- [ ] Uterus / Vagina (Reproductive)

- [ ] Skin

- [ ] Other

Mark all the places on the diagram below that you are experiencing pain, discomfort, and/or skin changes:

Front

Back

Notes

Daily Wellness Log

Date: ....   S   M   T   W   Th   F   Sa

Weight:
Temperature:

Hours of Sleep

0   1   2   3   4   5   6   7   8   9   10   11   12+

Sleep Quality

☆ ☆ ☆ ☆ ☆

Weather

- [ ] Sunny
- [ ] Partly Cloudy
- [ ] Cloudy
- [ ] Windy
- [ ] Stormy
- [ ] Light Rain
- [ ] Heavy Rain
- [ ] Light Snow
- [ ] Heavy Snow
- [ ] Other ....

Mood

- [ ] Happy
- [ ] Calm
- [ ] Confident
- [ ] Excited
- [ ] Loving
- [ ] Other ....
- [ ] Sad
- [ ] Angry
- [ ] Anxious
- [ ] Stressed
- [ ] Self-Critical
- [ ] Tired

Temperature

- [ ] Hot
- [ ] Warm
- [ ] Cold
- [ ] Damp
- [ ] Comfortable

Water

Energy Level

☆ ☆ ☆ ☆ ☆

Moon

- [ ] New Moon
- [ ] Waxing Crescent
- [ ] First Quarter
- [ ] Waxing Gibbous
- [ ] Full Moon
- [ ] Waning Gibbous
- [ ] Third Quarter
- [ ] Waning Crescent

Bowel Movement

Constipation   *Diarrhea*

Type 1	Type 2	Type 3	Type 4	Type 5	Type 6	Type 7

Medications

Time	Description

Vitamins

Time	Description

Exercise

Time	Intensity	Activity

Breakfast

Lunch

Dinner

Snacks

Menstrual Cycle Symptoms

- [ ] Cramps
- [ ] Headache
- [ ] Backache
- [ ] Nausea
- [ ] Fatigue
- [ ] Tender Breasts
- [ ] Acne
- [ ] Bloating
- [ ] Cravings
- [ ] Insomnia
- [ ] Other

Physical Symptoms Log

Period

- [ ] Spotting
- [ ] Light
- [ ] Medium
- [ ] Heavy

Pain, Discomfort and Skin Changes

(See the Pain Level Reference and/or Glossary for help in describing your symptoms)

Describe your symptoms, pain level and approximate time in the appropriate space below:

- [ ] Head / Ears / Eyes / Nose / Mouth

- [ ] Throat / Neck

- [ ] Shoulders / Arms / Hands

- [ ] Chest / Heart

- [ ] Back

- [ ] Hips / Buttocks / Legs / Feet

- [ ] Lungs / Breathing (Respiratory)

- [ ] Stomach / Abdomen (Digestive)

- [ ] Uterus / Vagina (Reproductive)

- [ ] Skin

- [ ] Other

Mark all the places on the diagram below that you are experiencing pain, discomfort, and/or skin changes:

Front

Back

Notes

Daily Wellness Log

Date: _____   S   M   T   W   Th   F   Sa

Weight: _____
Temperature: _____

Hours of Sleep

0   1   2   3   4   5   6   7   8   9   10   11   12+

Sleep Quality

☆ ☆ ☆ ☆ ☆

Weather

- [ ] Sunny ☀
- [ ] Partly Cloudy ☁
- [ ] Cloudy ⛅
- [ ] Windy 🌫
- [ ] Stormy ⛈
- [ ] Light Rain 🌧
- [ ] Heavy Rain 🌧
- [ ] Light Snow 🌨
- [ ] Heavy Snow 🌨
- [ ] Other _____

Mood

- [ ] Happy ☺
- [ ] Calm ☺
- [ ] Confident 😎
- [ ] Excited 😄
- [ ] Loving 😍
- [ ] Other
- [ ] Sad ☹
- [ ] Angry 😠
- [ ] Anxious 😟
- [ ] Stressed 😣
- [ ] Self-Critical 😡
- [ ] Tired 😫

Temperature

- [ ] Hot
- [ ] Warm
- [ ] Cold
- [ ] Damp
- [ ] Comfortable

Water

🥛 🥛 🥛 🥛 🥛 🥛 🥛 🥛

Energy Level

☆ ☆ ☆ ☆ ☆

Moon

- [ ] New Moon ●
- [ ] Waxing Crescent ●
- [ ] First Quarter ◑
- [ ] Waxing Gibbous ◑
- [ ] Full Moon ○
- [ ] Waning Gibbous ◐
- [ ] Third Quarter ◐
- [ ] Waning Crescent ◐

Bowel Movement

Constipation   *Diarrhea*

Type 1	Type 2	Type 3	Type 4	Type 5	Type 6	Type 7

Medications

Time	Description

Vitamins

Time	Description

Exercise

Time	Intensity	Activity

Breakfast

Lunch

Dinner

Snacks

Menstrual Cycle Symptoms

- [ ] Cramps
- [ ] Headache
- [ ] Backache
- [ ] Nausea
- [ ] Fatigue
- [ ] Tender Breasts
- [ ] Acne
- [ ] Bloating
- [ ] Cravings
- [ ] Insomnia
- [ ] Other

Physical Symptoms Log

Period

- [ ] Spotting
- [ ] Light
- [ ] Medium
- [ ] Heavy

Pain, Discomfort and Skin Changes

(See the Pain Level Reference and/or Glossary for help in describing your symptoms)

Describe your symptoms, pain level and approximate time in the appropriate space below:

- [ ] Head / Ears / Eyes / Nose / Mouth

- [ ] Throat / Neck

- [ ] Shoulders / Arms / Hands

- [ ] Chest / Heart

- [ ] Back

- [ ] Hips / Buttocks / Legs / Feet

- [ ] Lungs / Breathing (Respiratory)

- [ ] Stomach / Abdomen (Digestive)

- [ ] Uterus / Vagina (Reproductive)

- [ ] Skin

- [ ] Other

Mark all the places on the diagram below that you are experiencing pain, discomfort, and/or skin changes:

Front

Back

Notes

Daily Wellness Log

Date: ....   S   M   T   W   Th   F   Sa

Weight:
Temperature:

Hours of Sleep

0   1   2   3   4   5   6   7   8   9   10   11   12+

Sleep Quality

☆ ☆ ☆ ☆ ☆

Weather

- [ ] Sunny ☀
- [ ] Partly Cloudy ☁
- [ ] Cloudy ⛅
- [ ] Windy 🌬
- [ ] Stormy ⛈
- [ ] Light Rain 🌧
- [ ] Heavy Rain 🌧
- [ ] Light Snow 🌨
- [ ] Heavy Snow ❄
- [ ] Other ....

Mood

- [ ] Happy ☺
- [ ] Calm ☺
- [ ] Confident 😎
- [ ] Excited 😀
- [ ] Loving 😍
- [ ] Other
- [ ] Sad ☹
- [ ] Angry 😠
- [ ] Anxious 😧
- [ ] Stressed 😖
- [ ] Self-Critical 😤
- [ ] Tired 😫

Temperature

- [ ] Hot
- [ ] Warm
- [ ] Cold
- [ ] Damp
- [ ] Comfortable

Water

🥤 🥤 🥤 🥤 🥤 🥤 🥤 🥤

Energy Level

☆ ☆ ☆ ☆ ☆

Moon

- [ ] New Moon
- [ ] Waxing Crescent
- [ ] First Quarter
- [ ] Waxing Gibbous
- [ ] Full Moon
- [ ] Waning Gibbous
- [ ] Third Quarter
- [ ] Waning Crescent

Bowel Movement

Constipation   *Diarrhea*

Type 1	Type 2	Type 3	Type 4	Type 5	Type 6	Type 7

Medication

Time	Description

Vitamins

Time	Description

Exercise

Time	Intensity	Activity

Breakfast

Lunch

Dinner

Snacks

Menstrual Cycle Symptoms

- [ ] Cramps
- [ ] Headache
- [ ] Backache
- [ ] Nausea
- [ ] Fatigue
- [ ] Tender Breasts
- [ ] Acne
- [ ] Bloating
- [ ] Cravings
- [ ] Insomnia
- [ ] Other

Physical Symptoms Log

Period

- [ ] Spotting
- [ ] Light
- [ ] Medium
- [ ] Heavy

Pain, Discomfort and Skin Changes

(See the Pain Level Reference and/or Glossary for help in describing your symptoms)

Describe your symptoms, pain level and approximate time in the appropriate space below:

- [ ] Head / Ears / Eyes / Nose / Mouth

- [ ] Throat / Neck

- [ ] Shoulders / Arms / Hands

- [ ] Chest / Heart

- [ ] Back

- [ ] Hips / Buttocks / Legs / Feet

- [ ] Lungs / Breathing (Respiratory)

- [ ] Stomach / Abdomen (Digestive)

- [ ] Uterus / Vagina (Reproductive)

- [ ] Skin

- [ ] Other

Mark all the places on the diagram below that you are experiencing pain, discomfort, and/or skin changes:

Front

Back

Notes

Daily Wellness Log

Date: ....

S M T W Th F Sa

Weight:
Temperature:

Hours of Sleep
0 1 2 3 4 5 6 7 8 9 10 11 12+

Sleep Quality
☆ ☆ ☆ ☆ ☆

Weather
- [ ] Sunny ☀
- [ ] Partly Cloudy ☁
- [ ] Cloudy ⛅
- [ ] Windy 🌬
- [ ] Stormy ⛈
- [ ] Light Rain 🌦
- [ ] Heavy Rain 🌧
- [ ] Light Snow 🌨
- [ ] Heavy Snow 🌨
- [ ] Other ....

Mood
- [ ] Happy 🙂
- [ ] Calm 🙂
- [ ] Confident 😎
- [ ] Excited 😃
- [ ] Loving 😍
- [ ] Other
- [ ] Sad ☹
- [ ] Angry 😠
- [ ] Anxious 😕
- [ ] Stressed 😣
- [ ] Self-Critical 😡
- [ ] Tired 😫

Temperature
- [ ] Hot
- [ ] Warm
- [ ] Cold
- [ ] Damp
- [ ] Comfortable

Water
🥛 🥛 🥛 🥛 🥛 🥛 🥛 🥛

Energy Level
☆ ☆ ☆ ☆ ☆

Moon
- [ ] New Moon ●
- [ ] Waxing Crescent ●
- [ ] First Quarter ◑
- [ ] Waxing Gibbous ◑
- [ ] Full Moon ○
- [ ] Waning Gibbous ◐
- [ ] Third Quarter ◐
- [ ] Waning Crescent ●

Bowel Movement

Constipation   *Diarrhea*

Type 1	Type 2	Type 3	Type 4	Type 5	Type 6	Type 7

Medications

Time	Description

Vitamins

Time	Description

Exercise

Time	Intensity	Activity

Breakfast

Lunch

Dinner

Snacks

Menstrual Cycle Symptoms

- [ ] Cramps
- [ ] Headache
- [ ] Backache
- [ ] Nausea
- [ ] Fatigue
- [ ] Tender Breasts
- [ ] Acne
- [ ] Bloating
- [ ] Cravings
- [ ] Insomnia
- [ ] Other

Physical Symptoms Log

Period

- [ ] Spotting
- [ ] Light
- [ ] Medium
- [ ] Heavy

Pain, Discomfort and Skin Changes

(See the Pain Level Reference and/or Glossary for help in describing your symptoms)

Describe your symptoms, pain level and approximate time in the appropriate space below:

- [ ] Head / Ears / Eyes / Nose / Mouth

_____
_____
_____

- [ ] Throat / Neck

_____
_____
_____

- [ ] Shoulders / Arms / Hands

_____
_____
_____

- [ ] Chest / Heart

_____
_____
_____

- [ ] Back

_____
_____
_____

- [ ] Hips / Buttocks / Legs / Feet

_____
_____
_____

- [ ] Lungs / Breathing (Respiratory)

_____
_____
_____

- [ ] Stomach / Abdomen (Digestive)

_____
_____
_____

- [ ] Uterus / Vagina (Reproductive)

_____
_____
_____

- [ ] Skin

_____
_____
_____

- [ ] Other

_____
_____
_____

Mark all the places on the diagram below that you are experiencing pain, discomfort, and/or skin changes:

Front

Back

Notes

_____
_____
_____
_____

Daily Wellness Log

Date: ....   S M T W Th F Sa

Weight:
Temperature:

Hours of Sleep

0 1 2 3 4 5 6 7 8 9 10 11 12+

Sleep Quality
☆☆☆☆☆

Weather

- ☐ Sunny ☀
- ☐ Partly Cloudy ☁
- ☐ Cloudy ⛅
- ☐ Windy 🌫
- ☐ Stormy ⛈
- ☐ Light Rain 🌦
- ☐ Heavy Rain 🌧
- ☐ Light Snow 🌨
- ☐ Heavy Snow 🌨
- ☐ Other ....

Mood

- ☐ Happy ☺
- ☐ Calm ☺
- ☐ Confident 😎
- ☐ Excited 😄
- ☐ Loving 😍
- ☐ Other
- ☐ Sad ☹
- ☐ Angry 😠
- ☐ Anxious 😰
- ☐ Stressed 😣
- ☐ Self-Critical 😡
- ☐ Tired 😫

Temperature

☐ Hot ☐ Warm ☐ Cold ☐ Damp ☐ Comfortable

Water
🥤🥤🥤🥤🥤🥤🥤🥤

Energy Level
☆☆☆☆☆

Moon

- ☐ New Moon ●
- ☐ Waxing Crescent ●
- ☐ First Quarter ◑
- ☐ Waxing Gibbous ◑
- ☐ Full Moon ○
- ☐ Waning Gibbous ◐
- ☐ Third Quarter ◐
- ☐ Waning Crescent ◐

Bowel Movement

Constipation   *Diarrhea*

Type 1   Type 2   Type 3   Type 4   Type 5   Type 6   Type 7

Medications

Time	Description

Vitamins

Time	Description

Exercise

Time	Intensity	Activity

Breakfast

Lunch

Dinner

Snacks

Menstrual Cycle Symptoms

☐ Cramps　☐ Headache　☐ Backache　☐ Nausea　☐ Fatigue

☐ Tender Breasts　☐ Acne　☐ Bloating　☐ Cravings　☐ Insomnia

☐ Other

Physical Symptoms Log

Period

☐ Spotting　☐ Light　☐ Medium　☐ Heavy

Pain, Discomfort and Skin Changes

(See the Pain Level Reference and/or Glossary for help in describing your symptoms)

Describe your symptoms, pain level and approximate time in the appropriate space below:

☐ Head / Ears / Eyes / Nose / Mouth

_____
_____

☐ Throat / Neck

_____
_____

☐ Shoulders / Arms / Hands

_____
_____

☐ Chest / Heart

_____
_____

☐ Back

_____
_____

☐ Hips / Buttocks / Legs / Feet

_____
_____

☐ Lungs / Breathing (Respiratory)

_____
_____

☐ Stomach / Abdomen (Digestive)

_____
_____

☐ Uterus / Vagina (Reproductive)

_____
_____

☐ Skin

_____
_____

☐ Other

_____
_____

Mark all the places on the diagram below that you are experiencing pain, discomfort, and/or skin changes:

Front

Back

Notes
_____
_____
_____
_____

Daily Wellness Log

Date: ....   S M T W Th F Sa

Weight: _____
Temperature: _____

Hours of Sleep

0 1 2 3 4 5 6 7 8 9 10 11 12+

Sleep Quality

☆ ☆ ☆ ☆ ☆

Weather

- [ ] Sunny ☀
- [ ] Partly Cloudy ☁
- [ ] Cloudy ⛅
- [ ] Windy 🌬
- [ ] Stormy ⛈
- [ ] Light Rain 🌦
- [ ] Heavy Rain 🌧
- [ ] Light Snow 🌨
- [ ] Heavy Snow 🌨
- [ ] Other

Mood

- [ ] Happy 🙂
- [ ] Calm 🙂
- [ ] Confident 😎
- [ ] Excited 😀
- [ ] Loving 😍
- [ ] Other

- [ ] Sad ☹
- [ ] Angry 😠
- [ ] Anxious 😟
- [ ] Stressed 😣
- [ ] Self-Critical 😤
- [ ] Tired 😫

Temperature

- [ ] Hot
- [ ] Warm
- [ ] Cold
- [ ] Damp
- [ ] Comfortable

Water

🥛 🥛 🥛 🥛 🥛 🥛 🥛 🥛

Energy Level

☆ ☆ ☆ ☆ ☆

Moon

- [ ] New Moon ●
- [ ] Waxing Crescent ◗
- [ ] First Quarter ◑
- [ ] Waxing Gibbous ◐
- [ ] Full Moon ○
- [ ] Waning Gibbous ◑
- [ ] Third Quarter ◑
- [ ] Waning Crescent ◖

Bowel Movement

Constipation   *Diarrhea*

Type 1	Type 2	Type 3	Type 4	Type 5	Type 6	Type 7

Medications

Time	Description

Vitamins

Time	Description

Exercise

Time	Intensity	Activity

Breakfast

Lunch

Dinner

Snacks

Menstrual Cycle Symptoms

- [ ] Cramps
- [ ] Headache
- [ ] Backache
- [ ] Nausea
- [ ] Fatigue
- [ ] Tender Breasts
- [ ] Acne
- [ ] Bloating
- [ ] Cravings
- [ ] Insomnia
- [ ] Other

Physical Symptoms Log

Period

- [ ] Spotting
- [ ] Light
- [ ] Medium
- [ ] Heavy

Pain, Discomfort and Skin Changes

(See the Pain Level Reference and/or Glossary for help in describing your symptoms)

Describe your symptoms, pain level and approximate time in the appropriate space below:

- [ ] Head / Ears / Eyes / Nose / Mouth
- [ ] Throat / Neck
- [ ] Shoulders / Arms / Hands
- [ ] Chest / Heart
- [ ] Back
- [ ] Hips / Buttocks / Legs / Feet
- [ ] Lungs / Breathing (Respiratory)
- [ ] Stomach / Abdomen (Digestive)
- [ ] Uterus / Vagina (Reproductive)
- [ ] Skin
- [ ] Other

Mark all the places on the diagram below that you are experiencing pain, discomfort, and/or skin changes:

Front

Back

Notes

Daily Wellness Log

Date: ....

S M T W Th F Sa

Weight:
Temperature:

Hours of Sleep

0 1 2 3 4 5 6 7 8 9 10 11 12+

Sleep Quality

☆ ☆ ☆ ☆ ☆

Weather

- [ ] Sunny
- [ ] Partly Cloudy
- [ ] Cloudy
- [ ] Windy
- [ ] Stormy
- [ ] Light Rain
- [ ] Heavy Rain
- [ ] Light Snow
- [ ] Heavy Snow
- [ ] Other

Mood

- [ ] Happy
- [ ] Calm
- [ ] Confident
- [ ] Excited
- [ ] Loving
- [ ] Other
- [ ] Sad
- [ ] Angry
- [ ] Anxious
- [ ] Stressed
- [ ] Self-Critical
- [ ] Tired

Temperature

- [ ] Hot
- [ ] Warm
- [ ] Cold
- [ ] Damp
- [ ] Comfortable

Water

Energy Level

☆ ☆ ☆ ☆ ☆

Moon

- [ ] New Moon
- [ ] Waxing Crescent
- [ ] First Quarter
- [ ] Waxing Gibbous
- [ ] Full Moon
- [ ] Waning Gibbous
- [ ] Third Quarter
- [ ] Waning Crescent

Bowel Movement

Constipation   *Diarrhea*

Type 1	Type 2	Type 3	Type 4	Type 5	Type 6	Type 7

Medications

Time	Description

Vitamins

Time	Description

Exercise

Time	Intensity	Activity

Breakfast

Lunch

Dinner

Snacks

Menstrual Cycle Symptoms

- [ ] Cramps
- [ ] Headache
- [ ] Backache
- [ ] Nausea
- [ ] Fatigue
- [ ] Tender Breasts
- [ ] Acne
- [ ] Bloating
- [ ] Cravings
- [ ] Insomnia
- [ ] Other

Physical Symptoms Log

Period

- [ ] Spotting
- [ ] Light
- [ ] Medium
- [ ] Heavy

Pain, Discomfort and Skin Changes

(See the Pain Level Reference and/or Glossary for help in describing your symptoms)

Describe your symptoms, pain level and approximate time in the appropriate space below:

- [ ] Head / Ears / Eyes / Nose / Mouth

- [ ] Throat / Neck

- [ ] Shoulders / Arms / Hands

- [ ] Chest / Heart

- [ ] Back

- [ ] Hips / Buttocks / Legs / Feet

- [ ] Lungs / Breathing (Respiratory)

- [ ] Stomach / Abdomen (Digestive)

- [ ] Uterus / Vagina (Reproductive)

- [ ] Skin

- [ ] Other

Mark all the places on the diagram below that you are experiencing pain, discomfort, and/or skin changes:

Front

Back

Notes

Daily Wellness Log

Date: _____   S M T W Th F Sa

Weight: _____
Temperature: _____

Hours of Sleep

0 1 2 3 4 5 6 7 8 9 10 11 12+

Sleep Quality

☆ ☆ ☆ ☆ ☆

Weather

- [ ] Sunny ☀
- [ ] Partly Cloudy ⛅
- [ ] Cloudy ⛅
- [ ] Windy 🌬
- [ ] Stormy ⛈
- [ ] Light Rain 🌦
- [ ] Heavy Rain 🌧
- [ ] Light Snow 🌨
- [ ] Heavy Snow 🌨
- [ ] Other _____

Mood

- [ ] Happy ☺
- [ ] Calm ☺
- [ ] Confident 😎
- [ ] Excited 😃
- [ ] Loving 😍
- [ ] Other _____
- [ ] Sad ☹
- [ ] Angry 😠
- [ ] Anxious 😨
- [ ] Stressed 😣
- [ ] Self-Critical 😤
- [ ] Tired 😫

Temperature

- [ ] Hot
- [ ] Warm
- [ ] Cold
- [ ] Damp
- [ ] Comfortable

Water

☐ ☐ ☐ ☐ ☐ ☐ ☐ ☐

Energy Level

☆ ☆ ☆ ☆ ☆

Moon

- [ ] New Moon ●
- [ ] Waxing Crescent ●
- [ ] First Quarter ◑
- [ ] Waxing Gibbous ◑
- [ ] Full Moon ○
- [ ] Waning Gibbous ◐
- [ ] Third Quarter ◐
- [ ] Waning Crescent ◐

Bowel Movement

Constipation   *Diarrhea*

Type 1	Type 2	Type 3	Type 4	Type 5	Type 6	Type 7

Medication

Time	Description

Vitamins

Time	Description

Exercise

Time	Intensity	Activity

Breakfast

Lunch

Dinner

Snacks

Menstrual Cycle Symptoms

☐ Cramps ☐ Headache ☐ Backache ☐ Nausea ☐ Fatigue

☐ Tender Breasts ☐ Acne ☐ Bloating ☐ Cravings ☐ Insomnia

☐ Other

Physical Symptoms Log

Period

☐ Spotting ☐ Light ☐ Medium ☐ Heavy

Pain, Discomfort and Skin Changes

(See the Pain Level Reference and/or Glossary for help in describing your symptoms)

Describe your symptoms, pain level and approximate time in the appropriate space below:

☐ Head / Ears / Eyes / Nose / Mouth

☐ Throat / Neck

☐ Shoulders / Arms / Hands

☐ Chest / Heart

☐ Back

☐ Hips / Buttocks / Legs / Feet

☐ Lungs / Breathing (Respiratory)

☐ Stomach / Abdomen (Digestive)

☐ Uterus / Vagina (Reproductive)

☐ Skin

☐ Other

Mark all the places on the diagram below that you are experiencing pain, discomfort, and/or skin changes:

Front

Back

Notes

Daily Wellness Log

Date: ....   S M T W Th F Sa

Weight:
Temperature:

Hours of Sleep

0 1 2 3 4 5 6 7 8 9 10 11 12+

Sleep Quality

☆ ☆ ☆ ☆ ☆

Weather

- [ ] Sunny ☀
- [ ] Partly Cloudy ☁
- [ ] Cloudy ⛅
- [ ] Windy 🌬
- [ ] Stormy ⛈
- [ ] Light Rain 🌦
- [ ] Heavy Rain 🌧
- [ ] Light Snow 🌨
- [ ] Heavy Snow 🌨
- [ ] Other ....

Mood

- [ ] Happy ☺
- [ ] Calm ☺
- [ ] Confident 😎
- [ ] Excited 😃
- [ ] Loving 😍
- [ ] Other
- [ ] Sad ☹
- [ ] Angry 😠
- [ ] Anxious 😟
- [ ] Stressed 😖
- [ ] Self-Critical 😡
- [ ] Tired 😫

Temperature

- [ ] Hot
- [ ] Warm
- [ ] Cold
- [ ] Damp
- [ ] Comfortable

Water

⊔ ⊔ ⊔ ⊔ ⊔ ⊔ ⊔ ⊔

Energy Level

☆ ☆ ☆ ☆ ☆

Moon

- [ ] New Moon ●
- [ ] Waxing Crescent ◗
- [ ] First Quarter ◑
- [ ] Waxing Gibbous ◕
- [ ] Full Moon ○
- [ ] Waning Gibbous ◔
- [ ] Third Quarter ◐
- [ ] Waning Crescent ◖

Bowel Movement

Constipation   *Diarrhea*

Type 1	Type 2	Type 3	Type 4	Type 5	Type 6	Type 7

Medications

Time	Description

Vitamins

Time	Description

Exercise

Time	Intensity	Activity

Breakfast

Lunch

Dinner

Snacks

Menstrual Cycle Symptoms

☐ Cramps ☐ Headache ☐ Backache ☐ Nausea ☐ Fatigue

☐ Tender Breasts ☐ Acne ☐ Bloating ☐ Cravings ☐ Insomnia

☐ Other

Physical Symptoms Log

Period

☐ Spotting ☐ Light ☐ Medium ☐ Heavy

Pain, Discomfort and Skin Changes

(See the Pain Level Reference and/or Glossary for help in describing your symptoms)

Describe your symptoms, pain level and approximate time in the appropriate space below:

☐ Head / Ears / Eyes / Nose / Mouth

_____
_____
_____

☐ Throat / Neck

_____
_____

☐ Shoulders / Arms / Hands

_____
_____
_____

☐ Chest / Heart

_____
_____
_____

☐ Back

_____
_____
_____

☐ Hips / Buttocks / Legs / Feet

_____
_____
_____

☐ Lungs / Breathing (Respiratory)

_____
_____
_____

☐ Stomach / Abdomen (Digestive)

_____
_____
_____

☐ Uterus / Vagina (Reproductive)

_____
_____
_____

☐ Skin

_____
_____
_____

☐ Other

_____
_____

Mark all the places on the diagram below that you are experiencing pain, discomfort, and/or skin changes:

Front

Back

Notes

_____
_____
_____
_____

Daily Wellness Log

Date: _____   S M T W Th F Sa

Weight:
Temperature:

Hours of Sleep

0 1 2 3 4 5 6 7 8 9 10 11 12+

Sleep Quality
☆ ☆ ☆ ☆ ☆

Weather

- [ ] Sunny ☀
- [ ] Partly Cloudy ☁
- [ ] Cloudy ⛅
- [ ] Windy 🌬
- [ ] Stormy ⛈
- [ ] Light Rain 🌦
- [ ] Heavy Rain 🌧
- [ ] Light Snow 🌨
- [ ] Heavy Snow 🌨
- [ ] Other _____

Mood

- [ ] Happy 🙂
- [ ] Calm 🙂
- [ ] Confident 😎
- [ ] Excited 😃
- [ ] Loving 😍
- [ ] Other
- [ ] Sad ☹
- [ ] Angry 😠
- [ ] Anxious 😣
- [ ] Stressed 😖
- [ ] Self-Critical 😡
- [ ] Tired 😫

Temperature

- [ ] Hot   [ ] Warm   [ ] Cold   [ ] Damp   [ ] Comfortable

Water

🥛 🥛 🥛 🥛 🥛 🥛 🥛 🥛

Energy Level
☆ ☆ ☆ ☆ ☆

Moon

- [ ] New Moon ●
- [ ] Waxing Crescent ●
- [ ] First Quarter ◐
- [ ] Waxing Gibbous ◑
- [ ] Full Moon ○
- [ ] Waning Gibbous ◐
- [ ] Third Quarter ◑
- [ ] Waning Crescent ◑

Bowel Movement

Constipation   *Diarrhea*

Type 1	Type 2	Type 3	Type 4	Type 5	Type 6	Type 7

Medications

Time	Description

Vitamins

Time	Description

Exercise

Time	Intensity	Activity

Breakfast

Lunch

Dinner

Snacks

Menstrual Cycle Symptoms

☐ Cramps ☐ Headache ☐ Backache ☐ Nausea ☐ Fatigue

☐ Tender Breasts ☐ Acne ☐ Bloating ☐ Cravings ☐ Insomnia

☐ Other

Physical Symptoms Log

Period

☐ Spotting ☐ Light ☐ Medium ☐ Heavy

Pain, Discomfort and Skin Changes

(See the Pain Level Reference and/or Glossary for help in describing your symptoms)

Describe your symptoms, pain level and approximate time in the appropriate space below:

☐ Head / Ears / Eyes / Nose / Mouth

_____
_____
_____

☐ Throat / Neck

_____
_____

☐ Shoulders / Arms / Hands

_____
_____
_____

☐ Chest / Heart

_____
_____
_____

☐ Back

_____
_____
_____

☐ Hips / Buttocks / Legs / Feet

_____
_____

☐ Lungs / Breathing (Respiratory)

_____
_____
_____

☐ Stomach / Abdomen (Digestive)

_____
_____
_____

☐ Uterus / Vagina (Reproductive)

_____
_____
_____

☐ Skin

_____
_____
_____

☐ Other

_____
_____
_____

Mark all the places on the diagram below that you are experiencing pain, discomfort, and/or skin changes:

Front

Back

Notes

_____
_____
_____
_____

Daily Wellness Log

Date: ....   S M T W Th F Sa

Weight: _____
Temperature: _____

Hours of Sleep

0 1 2 3 4 5 6 7 8 9 10 11 12+

Sleep Quality

☆ ☆ ☆ ☆ ☆

Weather

- [ ] Sunny ☀
- [ ] Partly Cloudy ☁
- [ ] Cloudy ⛅
- [ ] Windy 🌬
- [ ] Stormy ⛈
- [ ] Light Rain 🌦
- [ ] Heavy Rain 🌧
- [ ] Light Snow 🌨
- [ ] Heavy Snow 🌨
- [ ] Other ....

Mood

- [ ] Happy ☺
- [ ] Calm ☺
- [ ] Confident 😎
- [ ] Excited 😀
- [ ] Loving 😍
- [ ] Other ....
- [ ] Sad ☹
- [ ] Angry 😠
- [ ] Anxious 😬
- [ ] Stressed 😣
- [ ] Self-Critical 😤
- [ ] Tired 😫

Temperature

- [ ] Hot
- [ ] Warm
- [ ] Cold
- [ ] Damp
- [ ] Comfortable

Water

⬜ ⬜ ⬜ ⬜ ⬜ ⬜ ⬜ ⬜

Energy Level

☆ ☆ ☆ ☆ ☆

Moon

- [ ] New Moon ●
- [ ] Waxing Crescent ◕
- [ ] First Quarter ◑
- [ ] Waxing Gibbous ◑
- [ ] Full Moon ○
- [ ] Waning Gibbous ◐
- [ ] Third Quarter ◐
- [ ] Waning Crescent ◑

Bowel Movement

Constipation   *Diarrhea*

Type 1	Type 2	Type 3	Type 4	Type 5	Type 6	Type 7

Medications

Time	Description

Vitamins

Time	Description

Exercise

Time	Intensity	Activity

Breakfast

Lunch

Dinner

Snacks

Menstrual Cycle Symptoms

- [ ] Cramps
- [ ] Headache
- [ ] Backache
- [ ] Nausea
- [ ] Fatigue
- [ ] Tender Breasts
- [ ] Acne
- [ ] Bloating
- [ ] Cravings
- [ ] Insomnia
- [ ] Other

Physical Symptoms Log

Period

- [ ] Spotting
- [ ] Light
- [ ] Medium
- [ ] Heavy

Pain, Discomfort and Skin Changes

(See the Pain Level Reference and/or Glossary for help in describing your symptoms)

Describe your symptoms, pain level and approximate time in the appropriate space below:

- [ ] Head / Ears / Eyes / Nose / Mouth

- [ ] Throat / Neck

- [ ] Shoulders / Arms / Hands

- [ ] Chest / Heart

- [ ] Back

- [ ] Hips / Buttocks / Legs / Feet

- [ ] Lungs / Breathing (Respiratory)

- [ ] Stomach / Abdomen (Digestive)

- [ ] Uterus / Vagina (Reproductive)

- [ ] Skin

- [ ] Other

Mark all the places on the diagram below that you are experiencing pain, discomfort, and/or skin changes:

Front

Back

Notes

Daily Wellness Log

Date: ....   S M T W Th F Sa

Weight: _____
Temperature: _____

Hours of Sleep

0 1 2 3 4 5 6 7 8 9 10 11 12+

Sleep Quality

☆ ☆ ☆ ☆ ☆

Weather

- ☐ Sunny ☀
- ☐ Partly Cloudy ☁
- ☐ Cloudy ⛅
- ☐ Windy
- ☐ Stormy ⛈
- ☐ Light Rain 🌧
- ☐ Heavy Rain 🌧
- ☐ Light Snow 🌨
- ☐ Heavy Snow 🌨
- ☐ Other

Mood

- ☐ Happy :)
- ☐ Calm :)
- ☐ Confident 😎
- ☐ Excited :)
- ☐ Loving 😍
- ☐ Other
- ☐ Sad ☹
- ☐ Angry 😠
- ☐ Anxious 😣
- ☐ Stressed 😣
- ☐ Self-Critical 😠
- ☐ Tired 😫

Temperature

☐ Hot   ☐ Warm   ☐ Cold   ☐ Damp   ☐ Comfortable

Water

🥛 🥛 🥛 🥛 🥛 🥛 🥛 🥛

Energy Level

☆ ☆ ☆ ☆ ☆

Moon

- ☐ New Moon ●
- ☐ Waxing Crescent ●
- ☐ First Quarter ◐
- ☐ Waxing Gibbous ◑
- ☐ Full Moon ○
- ☐ Waning Gibbous ◑
- ☐ Third Quarter ◑
- ☐ Waning Crescent ◐

Bowel Movement

Constipation   *Diarrhea*

Type 1   Type 2   Type 3   Type 4   Type 5   Type 6   Type 7

Medications

Time	Description

Vitamins

Time	Description

Exercise

Time	Intensity	Activity

Breakfast

Lunch

Dinner

Snacks

Menstrual Cycle Symptoms

- [ ] Cramps
- [ ] Headache
- [ ] Backache
- [ ] Nausea
- [ ] Fatigue
- [ ] Tender Breasts
- [ ] Acne
- [ ] Bloating
- [ ] Cravings
- [ ] Insomnia
- [ ] Other

Physical Symptoms Log

Period

- [ ] Spotting
- [ ] Light
- [ ] Medium
- [ ] Heavy

Pain, Discomfort and Skin Changes

(See the Pain Level Reference and/or Glossary for help in describing your symptoms)

Describe your symptoms, pain level and approximate time in the appropriate space below:

- [ ] Head / Ears / Eyes / Nose / Mouth

- [ ] Throat / Neck

- [ ] Shoulders / Arms / Hands

- [ ] Chest / Heart

- [ ] Back

- [ ] Hips / Buttocks / Legs / Feet

- [ ] Lungs / Breathing (Respiratory)

- [ ] Stomach / Abdomen (Digestive)

- [ ] Uterus / Vagina (Reproductive)

- [ ] Skin

- [ ] Other

Mark all the places on the diagram below that you are experiencing pain, discomfort, and/or skin changes:

Front

Back

Notes

Daily Wellness Log

Date: _____ S M T W Th F Sa

Weight: _____
Temperature: _____

Hours of Sleep

0   1   2   3   4   5   6   7   8   9   10   11   12+

Sleep Quality

☆ ☆ ☆ ☆ ☆

Weather

- ☐ Sunny ☀
- ☐ Partly Cloudy ☁
- ☐ Cloudy ⛅
- ☐ Windy 🌬
- ☐ Stormy ⛈
- ☐ Light Rain 🌦
- ☐ Heavy Rain 🌧
- ☐ Light Snow 🌨
- ☐ Heavy Snow 🌨
- ☐ Other

Mood

- ☐ Happy 🙂
- ☐ Calm 🙂
- ☐ Confident 😎
- ☐ Excited 😃
- ☐ Loving 😍
- ☐ Other
- ☐ Sad ☹
- ☐ Angry 😠
- ☐ Anxious 😦
- ☐ Stressed 😖
- ☐ Self-Critical 😡
- ☐ Tired 😫

Temperature

☐ Hot   ☐ Warm   ☐ Cold   ☐ Damp   ☐ Comfortable

Water

🥛 🥛 🥛 🥛 🥛 🥛 🥛 🥛

Energy Level

☆ ☆ ☆ ☆ ☆

Moon

- ☐ New Moon ●
- ☐ Waxing Crescent ◗
- ☐ First Quarter ◐
- ☐ Waxing Gibbous ◑
- ☐ Full Moon ○
- ☐ Waning Gibbous ◔
- ☐ Third Quarter ◑
- ☐ Waning Crescent ◑

Bowel Movement

Constipation   *Diarrhea*

Type 1	Type 2	Type 3	Type 4	Type 5	Type 6	Type 7

Medications

Time	Description

Vitamins

Time	Description

Exercise

Time	Intensity	Activity

Breakfast

Lunch

Dinner

Snacks

Menstrual Cycle Symptoms

- [ ] Cramps
- [ ] Headache
- [ ] Backache
- [ ] Nausea
- [ ] Fatigue
- [ ] Tender Breasts
- [ ] Acne
- [ ] Bloating
- [ ] Cravings
- [ ] Insomnia
- [ ] Other

Physical Symptoms Log

Period

- [ ] Spotting
- [ ] Light
- [ ] Medium
- [ ] Heavy

Pain, Discomfort and Skin Changes

(See the Pain Level Reference and/or Glossary for help in describing your symptoms)

Describe your symptoms, pain level and approximate time in the appropriate space below:

- [ ] Head / Ears / Eyes / Nose / Mouth

- [ ] Throat / Neck

- [ ] Shoulders / Arms / Hands

- [ ] Chest / Heart

- [ ] Back

- [ ] Hips / Buttocks / Legs / Feet

- [ ] Lungs / Breathing (Respiratory)

- [ ] Stomach / Abdomen (Digestive)

- [ ] Uterus / Vagina (Reproductive)

- [ ] Skin

- [ ] Other

Mark all the places on the diagram below that you are experiencing pain, discomfort, and/or skin changes:

Front

Back

Notes

Daily Wellness Log

Date: ....   S   M   T   W   Th   F   Sa

Weight:
Temperature:

Hours of Sleep

0   1   2   3   4   5   6   7   8   9   10   11   12+

Sleep Quality
☆ ☆ ☆ ☆ ☆

Weather

- [ ] Sunny ☀
- [ ] Partly Cloudy ☁
- [ ] Cloudy ⛅
- [ ] Windy 🌬
- [ ] Stormy ⛈
- [ ] Light Rain 🌦
- [ ] Heavy Rain 🌧
- [ ] Light Snow 🌨
- [ ] Heavy Snow 🌨
- [ ] Other ....

Mood

- [ ] Happy :)
- [ ] Calm :)
- [ ] Confident 😎
- [ ] Excited :D
- [ ] Loving 😍
- [ ] Other ....
- [ ] Sad :(
- [ ] Angry >:(
- [ ] Anxious :/
- [ ] Stressed >.<
- [ ] Self-Critical >:(
- [ ] Tired X(

Temperature

- [ ] Hot
- [ ] Warm
- [ ] Cold
- [ ] Damp
- [ ] Comfortable

Water
🥛 🥛 🥛 🥛 🥛 🥛 🥛 🥛

Energy Level
☆ ☆ ☆ ☆ ☆

Moon

- [ ] New Moon ●
- [ ] Waxing Crescent ◐
- [ ] First Quarter ◑
- [ ] Waxing Gibbous ◑
- [ ] Full Moon ○
- [ ] Waning Gibbous ◑
- [ ] Third Quarter ◑
- [ ] Waning Crescent ◑

Bowel Movement

Constipation   *Diarrhea*

Type 1	Type 2	Type 3	Type 4	Type 5	Type 6	Type 7

Medications

Time	Description

Vitamins

Time	Description

Exercise

Time	Intensity	Activity

Breakfast

Lunch

Dinner

Snacks

Menstrual Cycle Symptoms

- [ ] Cramps
- [ ] Headache
- [ ] Backache
- [ ] Nausea
- [ ] Fatigue
- [ ] Tender Breasts
- [ ] Acne
- [ ] Bloating
- [ ] Cravings
- [ ] Insomnia
- [ ] Other

Physical Symptoms Log

Period

- [ ] Spotting
- [ ] Light
- [ ] Medium
- [ ] Heavy

Pain, Discomfort and Skin Changes

(See the Pain Level Reference and/or Glossary for help in describing your symptoms)

Describe your symptoms, pain level and approximate time in the appropriate space below:

- [ ] Head / Ears / Eyes / Nose / Mouth
- [ ] Throat / Neck

- [ ] Shoulders / Arms / Hands
- [ ] Chest / Heart

- [ ] Back
- [ ] Hips / Buttocks / Legs / Feet

- [ ] Lungs / Breathing (Respiratory)
- [ ] Stomach / Abdomen (Digestive)

- [ ] Uterus / Vagina (Reproductive)
- [ ] Skin

- [ ] Other

Mark all the places on the diagram below that you are experiencing pain, discomfort, and/or skin changes:

Front

Back

Notes

Daily Wellness Log

Date: .... S M T W Th F Sa

Weight:

Temperature:

Hours of Sleep

0 1 2 3 4 5 6 7 8 9 10 11 12+

Sleep Quality

☆ ☆ ☆ ☆ ☆

Weather

- ☐ Sunny
- ☐ Partly Cloudy
- ☐ Cloudy
- ☐ Windy
- ☐ Stormy
- ☐ Light Rain
- ☐ Heavy Rain
- ☐ Light Snow
- ☐ Heavy Snow
- ☐ Other ....

Mood

- ☐ Happy
- ☐ Calm
- ☐ Confident
- ☐ Excited
- ☐ Loving
- ☐ Other
- ☐ Sad
- ☐ Angry
- ☐ Anxious
- ☐ Stressed
- ☐ Self-Critical
- ☐ Tired

Temperature

☐ Hot ☐ Warm ☐ Cold ☐ Damp ☐ Comfortable

Water

⊔ ⊔ ⊔ ⊔ ⊔ ⊔ ⊔ ⊔

Energy Level

☆ ☆ ☆ ☆ ☆

Moon

- ☐ New Moon
- ☐ Waxing Crescent
- ☐ First Quarter
- ☐ Waxing Gibbous
- ☐ Full Moon
- ☐ Waning Gibbous
- ☐ Third Quarter
- ☐ Waning Crescent

Bowel Movement

Constipation   *Diarrhea*

Type 1	Type 2	Type 3	Type 4	Type 5	Type 6	Type 7

Medications

Time	Description

Vitamins

Time	Description

Exercise

Time	Intensity	Activity

Breakfast

Lunch

Dinner

Snacks

Menstrual Cycle Symptoms

- [ ] Cramps
- [ ] Headache
- [ ] Backache
- [ ] Nausea
- [ ] Fatigue
- [ ] Tender Breasts
- [ ] Acne
- [ ] Bloating
- [ ] Cravings
- [ ] Insomnia
- [ ] Other

Physical Symptoms Log

Period

- [ ] Spotting
- [ ] Light
- [ ] Medium
- [ ] Heavy

Pain, Discomfort and Skin Changes

(See the Pain Level Reference and/or Glossary for help in describing your symptoms)

Describe your symptoms, pain level and approximate time in the appropriate space below:

- [ ] Head / Ears / Eyes / Nose / Mouth

- [ ] Throat / Neck

- [ ] Shoulders / Arms / Hands

- [ ] Chest / Heart

- [ ] Back

- [ ] Hips / Buttocks / Legs / Feet

- [ ] Lungs / Breathing (Respiratory)

- [ ] Stomach / Abdomen (Digestive)

- [ ] Uterus / Vagina (Reproductive)

- [ ] Skin

- [ ] Other

Mark all the places on the diagram below that you are experiencing pain, discomfort, and/or skin changes:

Front

Back

Notes

Daily Wellness Log

Date: _____   S M T W Th F Sa

Weight: _____

Temperature: _____

Hours of Sleep

0 1 2 3 4 5 6 7 8 9 10 11 12+

Sleep Quality

☆ ☆ ☆ ☆ ☆

Weather

- ☐ Sunny
- ☐ Partly Cloudy
- ☐ Cloudy
- ☐ Windy
- ☐ Stormy
- ☐ Light Rain
- ☐ Heavy Rain
- ☐ Light Snow
- ☐ Heavy Snow
- ☐ Other _____

Mood

- ☐ Happy
- ☐ Calm
- ☐ Confident
- ☐ Excited
- ☐ Loving
- ☐ Other _____
- ☐ Sad
- ☐ Angry
- ☐ Anxious
- ☐ Stressed
- ☐ Self-Critical
- ☐ Tired

Temperature

☐ Hot ☐ Warm ☐ Cold ☐ Damp ☐ Comfortable

Water

☐ ☐ ☐ ☐ ☐ ☐ ☐ ☐

Energy Level

☆ ☆ ☆ ☆ ☆

Moon

- ☐ New Moon
- ☐ Waxing Crescent
- ☐ First Quarter
- ☐ Waxing Gibbous
- ☐ Full Moon
- ☐ Waning Gibbous
- ☐ Third Quarter
- ☐ Waning Crescent

Bowel Movement

Constipation   Diarrhea

Type 1   Type 2   Type 3   Type 4   Type 5   Type 6   Type 7

Medications

Time	Description

Vitamins

Time	Description

Exercise

Time	Intensity	Activity

Breakfast

Lunch

Dinner

Snacks

Menstrual Cycle Symptoms

- ☐ Cramps
- ☐ Headache
- ☐ Backache
- ☐ Nausea
- ☐ Fatigue
- ☐ Tender Breasts
- ☐ Acne
- ☐ Bloating
- ☐ Cravings
- ☐ Insomnia
- ☐ Other

Physical Symptoms Log

Period

- ☐ Spotting
- ☐ Light
- ☐ Medium
- ☐ Heavy

Pain, Discomfort and Skin Changes

(See the Pain Level Reference and/or Glossary for help in describing your symptoms)

Describe your symptoms, pain level and approximate time in the appropriate space below:

☐ Head / Ears / Eyes / Nose / Mouth

_____

☐ Throat / Neck

_____

☐ Shoulders / Arms / Hands

_____

☐ Chest / Heart

_____

☐ Back

_____

☐ Hips / Buttocks / Legs / Feet

_____

☐ Lungs / Breathing (Respiratory)

_____

☐ Stomach / Abdomen (Digestive)

_____

☐ Uterus / Vagina (Reproductive)

_____

☐ Skin

_____

☐ Other

_____

Mark all the places on the diagram below that you are experiencing pain, discomfort, and/or skin changes:

Front

Back

Notes

_____

Daily Wellness Log

Date: ....   S M T W Th F Sa

Weight:
Temperature:

Hours of Sleep

0 1 2 3 4 5 6 7 8 9 10 11 12+

Sleep Quality
☆ ☆ ☆ ☆ ☆

Weather
- [ ] Sunny ☀
- [ ] Partly Cloudy ☁
- [ ] Cloudy ⛅
- [ ] Windy 🌫
- [ ] Stormy ⛈
- [ ] Light Rain 🌧
- [ ] Heavy Rain 🌧
- [ ] Light Snow 🌨
- [ ] Heavy Snow 🌨
- [ ] Other ....

Mood
- [ ] Happy 🙂
- [ ] Calm 🙂
- [ ] Confident 😎
- [ ] Excited 😄
- [ ] Loving 😎
- [ ] Other ....
- [ ] Sad ☹
- [ ] Angry 😠
- [ ] Anxious 😧
- [ ] Stressed 😖
- [ ] Self-Critical 😡
- [ ] Tired 😫

Temperature
- [ ] Hot
- [ ] Warm
- [ ] Cold
- [ ] Damp
- [ ] Comfortable

Water
▢ ▢ ▢ ▢ ▢ ▢ ▢

Energy Level
☆ ☆ ☆ ☆ ☆

Moon
- [ ] New Moon ●
- [ ] Waxing Crescent ●
- [ ] First Quarter ◐
- [ ] Waxing Gibbous ◑
- [ ] Full Moon ○
- [ ] Waning Gibbous ◔
- [ ] Third Quarter ◑
- [ ] Waning Crescent ◕

Bowel Movement

Constipation   *Diarrhea*

Type 1	Type 2	Type 3	Type 4	Type 5	Type 6	Type 7

Medications

Time	Description

Vitamins

Time	Description

Exercise

Time	Intensity	Activity

Breakfast

Lunch

Dinner

Snacks

Menstrual Cycle Symptoms

☐ Cramps ☐ Headache ☐ Backache ☐ Nausea ☐ Fatigue

☐ Tender Breasts ☐ Acne ☐ Bloating ☐ Cravings ☐ Insomnia

☐ Other

Physical Symptoms Log

Period

☐ Spotting ☐ Light ☐ Medium ☐ Heavy

Pain, Discomfort and Skin Changes

(See the Pain Level Reference and/or Glossary for help in describing your symptoms)

Describe your symptoms, pain level and approximate time in the appropriate space below:

☐ Head / Ears / Eyes / Nose / Mouth

_____

_____

☐ Shoulders / Arms / Hands

_____

_____

☐ Back

_____

_____

☐ Lungs / Breathing (Respiratory)

_____

_____

☐ Uterus / Vagina (Reproductive)

_____

_____

☐ Other

_____

_____

☐ Throat / Neck

_____

_____

☐ Chest / Heart

_____

_____

☐ Hips / Buttocks / Legs / Feet

_____

_____

☐ Stomach / Abdomen (Digestive)

_____

_____

☐ Skin

_____

_____

Mark all the places on the diagram below that you are experiencing pain, discomfort, and/or skin changes:

Front

Back

Notes

Daily Wellness Log

Date: ....   S M T W Th F Sa

Weight: ....
Temperature: ....

Hours of Sleep

0 1 2 3 4 5 6 7 8 9 10 11 12+

Sleep Quality
☆ ☆ ☆ ☆ ☆

Weather

- [ ] Sunny ☀
- [ ] Partly Cloudy ☁
- [ ] Cloudy ⛅
- [ ] Windy 🌬
- [ ] Stormy ⛈
- [ ] Light Rain 🌧
- [ ] Heavy Rain 🌧
- [ ] Light Snow 🌨
- [ ] Heavy Snow 🌨
- [ ] Other ....

Mood

- [ ] Happy ☺
- [ ] Calm ☺
- [ ] Confident 😎
- [ ] Excited ☺
- [ ] Loving 😍
- [ ] Other
- [ ] Sad ☹
- [ ] Angry 😠
- [ ] Anxious 😖
- [ ] Stressed 😣
- [ ] Self-Critical 😤
- [ ] Tired 😫

Temperature

- [ ] Hot
- [ ] Warm
- [ ] Cold
- [ ] Damp
- [ ] Comfortable

Water

🥛 🥛 🥛 🥛 🥛 🥛 🥛 🥛

Energy Level
☆ ☆ ☆ ☆ ☆

Moon

- [ ] New Moon ●
- [ ] Waxing Crescent ●
- [ ] First Quarter ◑
- [ ] Waxing Gibbous ◐
- [ ] Full Moon ○
- [ ] Waning Gibbous ◑
- [ ] Third Quarter ◑
- [ ] Waning Crescent ●

Bowel Movement

Constipation   *Diarrhea*

Type 1	Type 2	Type 3	Type 4	Type 5	Type 6	Type 7

Medications

Time	Description

Vitamins

Time	Description

Exercise

Time	Intensity	Activity

Breakfast

Lunch

Dinner

Snacks

Menstrual Cycle Symptoms

- ☐ Cramps
- ☐ Headache
- ☐ Backache
- ☐ Nausea
- ☐ Fatigue
- ☐ Tender Breasts
- ☐ Acne
- ☐ Bloating
- ☐ Cravings
- ☐ Insomnia
- ☐ Other

Physical Symptoms Log

Period

- ☐ Spotting
- ☐ Light
- ☐ Medium
- ☐ Heavy

Pain, Discomfort and Skin Changes

(See the Pain Level Reference and/or Glossary for help in describing your symptoms)

Describe your symptoms, pain level and approximate time in the appropriate space below:

☐ Head / Ears / Eyes / Nose / Mouth

☐ Throat / Neck

☐ Shoulders / Arms / Hands

☐ Chest / Heart

☐ Back

☐ Hips / Buttocks / Legs / Feet

☐ Lungs / Breathing (Respiratory)

☐ Stomach / Abdomen (Digestive)

☐ Uterus / Vagina (Reproductive)

☐ Skin

☐ Other

Mark all the places on the diagram below that you are experiencing pain, discomfort, and/or skin changes:

Front

Back

Notes

Daily Wellness Log

Date: ....

S   M   T   W   Th   F   Sa

Weight:
Temperature:

Hours of Sleep

0   1   2   3   4   5   6   7   8   9   10   11   12+

Sleep Quality
☆ ☆ ☆ ☆ ☆

Weather
- [ ] Sunny ☀
- [ ] Partly Cloudy ☁
- [ ] Cloudy ⛅
- [ ] Windy 🌬
- [ ] Stormy ⛈
- [ ] Light Rain 🌦
- [ ] Heavy Rain 🌧
- [ ] Light Snow 🌨
- [ ] Heavy Snow 🌨
- [ ] Other

Mood
- [ ] Happy 🙂
- [ ] Calm 🙂
- [ ] Confident 😎
- [ ] Excited 😃
- [ ] Loving 😍
- [ ] Other
- [ ] Sad 😟
- [ ] Angry 😠
- [ ] Anxious 😣
- [ ] Stressed 😫
- [ ] Self-Critical 😡
- [ ] Tired 😫

Temperature
- [ ] Hot
- [ ] Warm
- [ ] Cold
- [ ] Damp
- [ ] Comfortable

Water

Energy Level
☆ ☆ ☆ ☆ ☆

Moon
- [ ] New Moon ●
- [ ] Waxing Crescent ●
- [ ] First Quarter ◐
- [ ] Waxing Gibbous ◑
- [ ] Full Moon ○
- [ ] Waning Gibbous ◑
- [ ] Third Quarter ◑
- [ ] Waning Crescent ◐

Bowel Movement

Constipation   *Diarrhea*

Type 1	Type 2	Type 3	Type 4	Type 5	Type 6	Type 7

Medications

Time	Description

Vitamins

Time	Description

Exercise

Time	Intensity	Activity

Breakfast

Lunch

Dinner

Snacks

Menstrual Cycle Symptoms

- [ ] Cramps
- [ ] Headache
- [ ] Backache
- [ ] Nausea
- [ ] Fatigue
- [ ] Tender Breasts
- [ ] Acne
- [ ] Bloating
- [ ] Cravings
- [ ] Insomnia
- [ ] Other

Physical Symptoms Log

Period

- [ ] Spotting
- [ ] Light
- [ ] Medium
- [ ] Heavy

Pain, Discomfort and Skin Changes

(See the Pain Level Reference and/or Glossary for help in describing your symptoms)

Describe your symptoms, pain level and approximate time in the appropriate space below:

- [ ] Head / Ears / Eyes / Nose / Mouth

- [ ] Throat / Neck

- [ ] Shoulders / Arms / Hands

- [ ] Chest / Heart

- [ ] Back

- [ ] Hips / Buttocks / Legs / Feet

- [ ] Lungs / Breathing (Respiratory)

- [ ] Stomach / Abdomen (Digestive)

- [ ] Uterus / Vagina (Reproductive)

- [ ] Skin

- [ ] Other

Mark all the places on the diagram below that you are experiencing pain, discomfort, and/or skin changes:

Front

Back

Notes

Daily Wellness Log

Date: ....   S   M   T   W   Th   F   Sa

Weight:
Temperature:

Hours of Sleep

0   1   2   3   4   5   6   7   8   9   10   11   12+

Sleep Quality

☆ ☆ ☆ ☆ ☆

Weather

- [ ] Sunny
- [ ] Partly Cloudy
- [ ] Cloudy
- [ ] Windy
- [ ] Stormy
- [ ] Light Rain
- [ ] Heavy Rain
- [ ] Light Snow
- [ ] Heavy Snow
- [ ] Other

Mood

- [ ] Happy
- [ ] Calm
- [ ] Confident
- [ ] Excited
- [ ] Loving
- [ ] Other
- [ ] Sad
- [ ] Angry
- [ ] Anxious
- [ ] Stressed
- [ ] Self-Critical
- [ ] Tired

Temperature

- [ ] Hot   [ ] Warm   [ ] Cold   [ ] Damp   [ ] Comfortable

Water

Energy Level

☆ ☆ ☆ ☆ ☆

Moon

- [ ] New Moon
- [ ] Waxing Crescent
- [ ] First Quarter
- [ ] Waxing Gibbous
- [ ] Full Moon
- [ ] Waning Gibbous
- [ ] Third Quarter
- [ ] Waning Crescent

Bowel Movement

Constipation   *Diarrhea*

Type 1	Type 2	Type 3	Type 4	Type 5	Type 6	Type 7

Medications

Time	Description

Vitamins

Time	Description

Exercise

Time	Intensity	Activity

Breakfast

Lunch

Dinner

Snacks

Menstrual Cycle Symptoms

- [ ] Cramps
- [ ] Headache
- [ ] Backache
- [ ] Nausea
- [ ] Fatigue
- [ ] Tender Breasts
- [ ] Acne
- [ ] Bloating
- [ ] Cravings
- [ ] Insomnia
- [ ] Other

Physical Symptoms Log

Period

- [ ] Spotting
- [ ] Light
- [ ] Medium
- [ ] Heavy

Pain, Discomfort and Skin Changes

(See the Pain Level Reference and/or Glossary for help in describing your symptoms)

Describe your symptoms, pain level and approximate time in the appropriate space below:

- [ ] Head / Ears / Eyes / Nose / Mouth
- [ ] Throat / Neck
- [ ] Shoulders / Arms / Hands
- [ ] Chest / Heart
- [ ] Back
- [ ] Hips / Buttocks / Legs / Feet
- [ ] Lungs / Breathing (Respiratory)
- [ ] Stomach / Abdomen (Digestive)
- [ ] Uterus / Vagina (Reproductive)
- [ ] Skin
- [ ] Other

Mark all the places on the diagram below that you are experiencing pain, discomfort, and/or skin changes:

Front

Back

Notes

Daily Wellness Log

Date: ....   S M T W Th F Sa

Weight:

Temperature:

Hours of Sleep

0 1 2 3 4 5 6 7 8 9 10 11 12+

Sleep Quality

☆ ☆ ☆ ☆ ☆

Weather

- [ ] Sunny
- [ ] Partly Cloudy
- [ ] Cloudy
- [ ] Windy
- [ ] Stormy
- [ ] Light Rain
- [ ] Heavy Rain
- [ ] Light Snow
- [ ] Heavy Snow
- [ ] Other ....

Mood

- [ ] Happy
- [ ] Calm
- [ ] Confident
- [ ] Excited
- [ ] Loving
- [ ] Other ....
- [ ] Sad
- [ ] Angry
- [ ] Anxious
- [ ] Stressed
- [ ] Self-Critical
- [ ] Tired

Temperature

- [ ] Hot
- [ ] Warm
- [ ] Cold
- [ ] Damp
- [ ] Comfortable

Water

Energy Level

☆ ☆ ☆ ☆ ☆

Moon

- [ ] New Moon
- [ ] Waxing Crescent
- [ ] First Quarter
- [ ] Waxing Gibbous
- [ ] Full Moon
- [ ] Waning Gibbous
- [ ] Third Quarter
- [ ] Waning Crescent

Bowel Movement

Constipation   *Diarrhea*

Type 1	Type 2	Type 3	Type 4	Type 5	Type 6	Type 7

Medications

Time	Description

Vitamins

Time	Description

Exercise

Time	Intensity	Activity

Breakfast

Lunch

Dinner

Snacks

Menstrual Cycle Symptoms

☐ Cramps ☐ Headache ☐ Backache ☐ Nausea ☐ Fatigue

☐ Tender Breasts ☐ Acne ☐ Bloating ☐ Cravings ☐ Insomnia

☐ Other

Physical Symptoms Log

Period

☐ Spotting ☐ Light ☐ Medium ☐ Heavy

Pain, Discomfort and Skin Changes

(See the Pain Level Reference and/or Glossary for help in describing your symptoms)

Describe your symptoms, pain level and approximate time in the appropriate space below:

☐ Head / Ears / Eyes / Nose / Mouth

☐ Throat / Neck

☐ Shoulders / Arms / Hands

☐ Chest / Heart

☐ Back

☐ Hips / Buttocks / Legs / Feet

☐ Lungs / Breathing (Respiratory)

☐ Stomach / Abdomen (Digestive)

☐ Uterus / Vagina (Reproductive)

☐ Skin

☐ Other

Mark all the places on the diagram below that you are experiencing pain, discomfort, and/or skin changes:

Front

Back

Notes

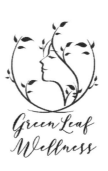

GreenLeaf
Wellness

Proudly made and designed in the U.S.A.

The material in this book is for informational purposes only and is not intended as
a substitute for the advice and care of your physician. Any person with a condition
requiring medical attention should consult a qualified medical practioner or therapist.
The author and publisher expressly disclaim responsibility for any adverse effects that
may result from the use or application of the information contained in this book.

Made in the USA
Coppell, TX
11 October 2021